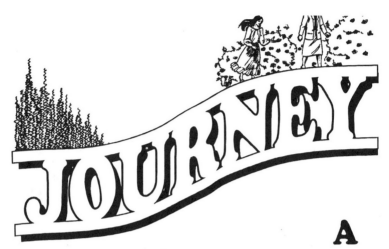

A BREAST CANCER SURVIVAL GUIDE

Allie Fair Sawyer
Norma Suzette Jones

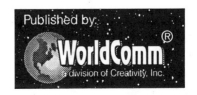

Published by:
WorldComm®
a division of Creativity, Inc.

Publisher: Ralph Roberts

Editor: Kathryn L. Hall

Cover Design: Melody Grandy Keller

Interior Design and Electronic Page Assembly: WorldComm®

Printed in the United States of America

10 9 8 7 6 5 4 3 2 1

ISBN 1-56664-012-1

WorldComm Press—a Division of Creativity, Inc., 65 Macedonia Road, Alexander, North Carolina 28701, (704) 252-9515—is a full service publisher.

Contents

ABOUT THIS BOOK. . .

Life *after* cancer--that's what this book is about. It's about dealing with the physical and emotional pain of the disease, it's about hope, it's about a fuller life as a result of the experience. The authors' willingness to share their innermost feelings shows that they have grown and that they are *free*--free to express emotion and free to be that unique individual that each of us is.

--Norma Messer, M.A.

This book is an inspiring testament given by two beautiful women. Through their initial descriptions of despair and doubt, you will be reminded of Job.

As you continue to read their story, you will be gently moved to writings of praise and hope—just as in the Psalms.

And finally, they share their wisdom, gathered from personal experiences and fact–searching research. You will be reminded of Proverbs.

This book will touch you, for you will become more sensitive to these important aspects of life—love and living.

--Dr. Daniel B. Veazey, M.D.

I believe that this book will share some insights and integral aspects of "full person healing" that simply cannot be taught in a physician's office. Here is a glimpse of the healing process that lies beyond office visits, radiation therapy, chemotherapy. . .

--Dr. Michael J. Zboyovski, Sr., D.C.

The authors of this book have "been through it" and have come out on top. The book is full of helpful facts and suggestions, and is also an engaging sharing of the authors and others' personal battles. I highly recommend it for anyone who has cancer, has had cancer, or has a family member with cancer.

--Marcia N. Davis, M.S.W., C.C.S.W.

INTRODUCTION

If this book will help, console, inspire, or touch the heart of even one woman who feels alone, fearful, or mutilated by breast cancer, it will fulfill its purpose.

The authors have given examples from personal experiences about problems unique to breast cancer survivors. Information about support groups, nutrition, emotional trials, fear of recurrence, medical treatments, clothing, lymphedema, humor, and much more, is included. All of the things which have been good therapy for the authors, hopefully will be good for the readers also.

This book is written for the thousands of women who will be diagnosed with breast cancer this year, and thousands more who are living in the aftermath of breast cancer and its treatments. It is the result of collaboration by two survivors. Two women who simply want to share with other women their feelings about the emotional and physical aspects of breast cancer. It is not their intent to be negative, to frighten, or to depress anyone. They know that only by being totally honest about their illness, treatments, pain, and fear can they continue their healing journey toward recovery. They cannot deny their emotions. When they feel the fear, the pain, and the hurt, they must deal with it in order to continue the healing process. The authors enjoy a very special friendship which began after their first meeting in a therapy support group. They represent very different life styles in many respects, and might never have known each other if they had not been brought together by the common bond of breast cancer.

ACKNOWLEDGEMENTS

I thank God for this second chance at Life. I thank my family and friends for standing by my side.

A very special thank you to some very special people:

To Elsie—I thank you for being there for me every step of the way. Even during the times when I was difficult to live with—you were there. You cared for me in the darkest times and provided hope by your presence. May your life be filled with joy!

To Karen—I thank you for your constant and continuous love and support, for the countless hours you spent with me at the hospital and during treatments. Thanks to John for being there for you.

To Angie and Chuck—although you were not geographically in the area, your frequent telephone calls and caring thoughts were close.

To Chris—I understand your fears, your pain, and your feelings of being alone. You dealt with these in your own way.

To my very dear friends Ann, Norma, Pat, Shirley, Dora, Rae, Edith, Thelma, Dale, Wanda, Linda, Ruby,

Loraine, Lynne, Lydia, and others—thanks for your love, support, and words of encouragement.

To my pastor, Rev. Aubrey Folk, for the frequent calls, visits, and prayers—you were a blessing.

To those gifted physicians, nurses, and health professionals who generously and patiently cared for me—I offer my gratitude.

To Dr. Lewis Rathbun and the Life After Cancer–Pathways counselors—Marcia, Norma, Peg, Jeannie, and Mary Ann, who gave so much of themselves; and to all the members of the support group for sharing and caring—I love and appreciate you!

—*Allie Fair Sawyer*

With love and gratitude, I thank the following important people: My husband, my children, my grandchildren, those family members and friends who helped, the leaders and members of the support groups I belong to, and the doctors, nurses, and other medical professionals who have been and are a part of my life.

—*Norma S. Jones*

Definition

. . .of a Cancer Survivor

Anyone with a history of cancer, from the time of diagnosis and for the remainder of life, whether that is for several months, years, or decades.

. . .of Cancer Survivorship

The concept of cancer survivorship affirms the potential of quality living after a cancer diagnosis and addresses those issues which affect that quality.

--National Coalition for Cancer Survivorship

A Letter of Good-bye to My Breast

I still, sometimes, feel you are a part of me—I reach to touch you, but you are gone.

To the ones who had to take you, you were only globs of fat and tissue and nerves and blood—for me, you had shape and warmth and softness and feeling and purpose.

It was such a shock to me that cancer could hide within you—you, so close to my heart and so much a part of my femininity.

Oh, some days, I'm adjusted to the reality that you are gone, but—even after all this time—I mourn you. I miss you.

I had to give up your warmth and beauty. I had to let go of you. I had to let you be destroyed—you were diseased. You might have killed me.

I say good-bye to you—forever. I will never again see you as a part of my body in this life. You had to be sacrificed so that I could have a better chance to go on living.

I cry for you often. Big crocodile tears of absolute sadness spill out of my eyes, roll down my face, and drip onto my chest—where once, you were.

—Norma

NORMA'S ROLLER COASTER RIDE

1989: My First Mastectomy

Being diagnosed with breast cancer started me on an emotional roller coaster ride, which zoomed out of control, with me along as a very reluctant and shocked passenger. It began in January of 1989. I was 41 years old, still married to my high school sweetheart, mother of two grown children, and celebrating the birth of my first grandchild. I definitely was not expecting to have the rug jerked out from under me in such an abrupt way.

I saw my family doctor in January of 1989 because I had a cold and was feeling extremely tired. While I was there, I asked him to feel a lump slightly above my right breast, below the collar bone. To me, it felt like a thick, flattened almond. I told him it felt very hot and that I thought I had pneumonia. After examining the lump, he said he didn't believe in waiting around, and scheduled me for a check-up with a surgeon that same week. I'll always be grateful for his quick and appropriate action.

The surgeon thought the lump might be a fibrocystic lump, but needed to do a biopsy to be sure. I had already had my most recent mammogram only six months earlier and wasn't the least bit fearful that this lump was anything serious. It was an extreme shock when the surgeon cut right into the little mass of cancer.

I knew something wasn't quite right when another surgeon in the office came in to assist. I was given more shots for pain and eventually fainted. They examined the biopsy sample there, then sent it across the street to the hospital lab for a frozen section to be done. With two experienced surgeons seeing the cancer, and the results of the microscopic test and frozen section examination by a pathologist, there was no doubt about what it was.

An estrogen receptor test of the biopsy sample was done at this time also. I was later to learn that because it was positive (meaning my estrogen fed the cancer), I would be taking tamoxifen, a hormone therapy drug used in treatment of this condition, for the next five years.

At this point, I had been revived and had been waiting for almost an hour to hear the results. I'll never forget the surgeon's words after he had asked me whether or not I was there alone. I told him I wasn't alone, and he said, "I'm sorry, but it is cancer, infiltrating ductal endemocarcinoma." Nothing registered but the word *cancer*, and I started crying.

During the days that followed, I went through all

the phases of denial, anger, fear, and self-pity that are generally associated with receiving such traumatic news. I felt a cold, stark fear which squeezed the breath from my lungs and made my heart skip every other beat. I felt so bewildered. I asked myself, *"Why me? What have I done to deserve this? Am I going to die? Please God, don't let me die! I have a lot to do, so many things I haven't finished, I don't want to leave all of these people that I love."*

And then, I felt angry. I was just so mad! At life, at fate, at everything, for letting this happen to me. The reality of having *cancer* just wouldn't sink in. It was more like a nightmare that kept replaying in my brain. I wanted to run away and hide in the hopes it would all go away, but I immediately discovered you can't run away from your own body. Finally, I accepted that it was true and knew I had to do something. *FAST!* I had choices to make, and my life literally depended on those choices.

I'm no quitter, so I made up my mind to meet this enemy called "Cancer" head-on. I was determined to fight for my life and win. This meant having my soft, warm breast cut away from my body. A modified radical mastectomy, with removal of all lymph nodes, was done a week after the biopsy in January, 1989. The lymph nodes were all negative of cancer and there was no more cancer in the breast. I did well after the surgery and went home after spending three days in the hospital.

Fighting cancer also meant having radiation sear

its way through my skin, bones, lungs, and nerve endings. (The radiation treatments, chemotherapy, and tamoxifen were all started during the same week in February of 1989—just three weeks after the surgery.) From then until August followed seven months of chemotherapy treatment, four of which were given during the five weeks of radiation. One week after the final radiation treatment, I developed lymphedema (permanent swelling) of my right arm and hand.

The chemotherapy drugs I received were cyclophosphamide (Cytoxan), methotrexate, and fluorouracil, commonly known as the *CMF protocol*. These drugs bloated my body with extra fluid, caused my hair and eyelashes to fall out, caused nausea and vomiting, diarrhea, mouth sores, and all in all, made me so sick and weak that I felt like I was walking through the halls of hell.

At this time, the newer drugs for nausea and vomiting were not available to me, or I would have had an easier time of it. I spent a lot of nights lying with a pillow and blanket on the bathroom floor because I was too sick to go to bed and sleep. I wretched so often during the first few days after each chemotherapy treatment that the blood vessels in my esophagus broke and I would have long red strings of blood and saliva hanging from my mouth. I felt, at times, like I was on fire, with sparks shooting from my hair and hot lava running through my veins. I was a "fire-breathing dragon." The oncologist finally decided just to keep me knocked out with drugs for the first couple of days after a treatment.

Four months after the mastectomy, I was put to sleep for a biopsy of my left breast. Several biopsies have followed since then, but that first one after the surgery and radiation, and during the chemo, was the worst.

Along with all of the physical problems came the emotional trauma. I felt like I was going down a busy interstate during rush hour on roller skates, as I became confused in a maze of medical jargon, terms, tests, machinery, needles, instructions, and medications. My nerves were shot and I had many, many sleepless nights as I struggled to make sane and important decisions.

Fighting my way through all of this pain and misery was made easier by my loving husband and children. They became valiant warriors in my ordeal and stood shoulder to shoulder with me to the end of the treatments. Other relatives and friends also gave much of their time and support to my immediate family and me during those long and difficult days of 1989.

I must admit, I wasn't a strong or brave warrior all of the time. I cried in my food. I cried in the shower, and when I got dressed. I cried when I went shopping (especially in lingerie departments), and I cried alone late at night. Those first few months, I cried a river of tears.

In the beginning, I felt very humiliated because I

was missing an important part of the physical me. I did feel like I had been mutilated by the amputation of my breast. My long-held (lifetime) image of myself, along with my self-respect, took a nose-dive every time I looked at my scarred body and my swollen hand and arm. Ending up with lymphedema or chronic swelling of my whole right arm and hand was another bucket of ice water thrown in my face!

Flashes of scenes stay with me. I remember my tears dropping in the plate of food in front of me many times. I see tears dropping into the bubbles of a nice warm bubble bath, or the tears running down my face to mingle with the water while showering. I remember standing outside on the porch, pulling my long hair out by the handfuls and letting the wind blow it away as I wondered, "Will a bird or some small animal use my silky hair to build part of its nest?"

During the first few months after my diagnosis of breast cancer, and during the treatments, I cried a lot. I cried for the part of me that was gone—my right breast. "My breast! My soft, warm breast. I want you back," I cried. "My arm. I want my real arm back. I want my old, strong, normal arm back," I cried.

But eventually, reality sinks in. You heal emotionally and are able to say, "I miss you Breast, but I'm glad you're gone from my body! I'll have a fighting chance without your cancer–filled form being a part of me. I'm sorry Arm that you are weak, swollen, and painful, but I'm glad you're still with me. I love you and I'll give you lots of TLC."

I must say that there were times when I was so sick and so depressed that I thought, "OK. I give up. Maybe it is time for me to die. I'll just go ahead and die. That will make it a lot easier on me and everybody else." But every time I had those thoughts, something, some tiny spark of something down deep in my soul, said "Hold on there a minute—you can't give up! You have the intelligence and the will and the strength to fight and survive! Don't you?" And so I began gathering all of the information that I thought might help me in this battle of a lifetime—the battle against cancer.

My Solutions

I discovered that one must have a basic and genuine love of *life* to put up a truly valiant struggle against cancer. As Kermit says, "It's not easy being green." And neither is it easy taking medicines and treatments which make you terribly sick in order to make you well. You wonder, at times when you are too weak to stand, if the cure really is better than the cause. Well, I'm here to tell you—the cure is worth it!

While on my never-ending journey of gathering information and seeking answers, I found a therapy support group in Asheville, North Carolina called Life After Cancer–Pathways. This marvelous group has changed my life for the better.

I have learned more about myself and about quality of life since 1990 than I ever thought possible. We have shared some very personal and gut-

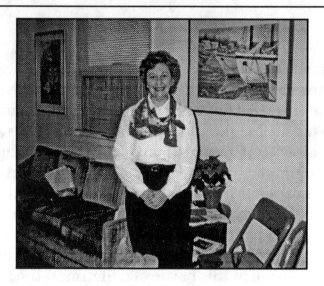

The co-author, Norma Suzette, shortly after her final mastectomy. She says, "I wasn't able to wear a bra or prosthesis yet, so I did creative things with scarves."

wrenching fears and experiences with each other in the group and this has helped our healing process go much faster. We have worked on the "inner child," letting go of hang-ups, fear of death, fear of a recurrence; we enhanced our belief in risk taking, the beauty of life, love of self and others; and we bettered our understanding of nutrition, relaxation, the latest medical technology, and other topics.

One of the things I have learned, for example, is that if I do have a recurrence of cancer and nothing in this world can be done to cure it—and I've done my best to beat it and can't—then it would be OK to die. To die does not mean one is a failure. This gives me a sense of peace—knowing that it's OK to die if my body is just too sick for me to stay in it any longer.

But hey, meanwhile, I'm very much alive and kicking. I didn't pay to ride on this roller coaster called cancer, and even though at times I wanted off of it desperately, I did survive the ride. I'll never be the same physically, but I've had a tremendous attitude adjustment and I'm happier mentally, emotionally, and spiritually.

I have inner peace, I have less stress, and I'm free to try new things. Believe me, getting to where I am now was no bed of roses. The emotional upheaval I have been through makes me appreciate each new day for just the day it is, and I have tons of love to give away.

Although being positive, taking the medicine (with its side effects), adjusting my attitude, and being health conscious is hard work, the rewards are great. I have learned so many things and stored so much new knowledge in my mind and soul, that I now have the ability (and the need) to let go of the sorrow, heartache, and depression I felt when I was first diagnosed and treated in 1989.

The fear that death has its icy cold grip on me has been replaced with new dignity, knowledge, hope, happiness, and peace. I am free of some of the old emotional baggage I carried around for years. I can better deal with pain and stress now, and I am putting the puzzle of myself back together with new and better puzzle pieces. I love my life, and I'm growing pretty fond of the idea that I am going to be around for many wonderful years to come, after all.

Of all the millions of homes in the world, not one has the same collection of items as mine. Of all the millions of people in the world, not one has the same collection of cells in their bodies as I have in mine. Of all the billions of thoughts in the world, not one person has exactly the same pattern of thoughts as I do. I am one of a kind. I am unique—just as you are.

My favorite colors are green, pink, and purple. I don't like liver. I do like asparagus. I have acrophobia (fear of heights), and am farsighted. I love my family and am devoted to their happiness. I like classical music. One of my favorite movies is *Gone With the Wind*. I like my rock garden and all semiprecious stones. I am an average woman, and I am a breast cancer survivor.

Having breast cancer hasn't changed my likes and dislikes totally, but now I am learning to appreciate some things I didn't like before. Those people I loved before, I now love more deeply and purely than words can describe.

Breast cancer isn't a death warrant. It's a disease you have, treat, get rid of, and then go on living. I didn't like breast cancer, but I really do love being alive. I have discovered (or maybe it's better to say *rediscovered*) that the spirit is most important of all, and that life really is very precious. I don't take anything or anyone in my life for granted. I have many plans for the future—many hopes and dreams.

I've got the rest of my life to give love to my family and friends and receive their love back. Isn't it nice to be loved! I like being me.

1991: My Second (and Last) Mastectomy

After surviving a modified radical mastectomy for breast cancer, five weeks of radiation from a linear accelerator, six months of CMF chemotherapy treatments, three years taking tamoxifen, and three years with lymphedema of my whole arm and hand, I decided to have a prophylactic simple mastectomy of my left breast in November of 1991 for the following reasons:

I was at high risk of developing cancer in the remaining breast because of the former cancer, which was a fast growing, infiltrating ductal carcinoma. Not only was the cancer arranged in tumors, but it was also sprinkled throughout the tissue in an individual cell fashion. Calcifications also had to be considered because they may sometimes become malignant.

There is a history of cancer, including breast cancer, on both sides of my family.

Also, I was developing more and more lumps in my remaining breast because of fibrocystic disease. This disease had plagued me since my first baseline mammogram at the age of 35. When you have a lot of these little fibrocystic lumps, shaped like dried beans or BB's, it's impossible to tell which one might be a bad guy unless you have a biopsy or other reliable tests. I was tired of biopsies because they are stress-ful, painful, and scarring.

I knew that if I did develop cancer in the remaining breast and had to have the same types of treatments as before, I might get lymphedema of my remaining "good" arm. The weight of the silicone prosthesis I wore on the right side aggravated the pain and swelling in my arm with lymphedema, forcing me to use a compression sleeve and glove, and also a sequential pneumatic arm pump more often.

I felt lopsided and wanted to feel even. Each woman deals with the problem of body-image after breast cancer surgery in her own way. Each woman has her own choices to make, and this is the way I felt then. I may change my mind in the future about implants as newer and better technology becomes available, but for now, I am satisfied with the way I look.

I was tired of worrying about the unknown and knew I would feel safer with some of that stress gone. Having a simple mastectomy of the remaining breast has decreased the risk of a recurrence and increased my chances for a longer, healthier life. The *quality* of life is now much more important to me than the *quantity*.

I went into the last mastectomy of my life with three years of experience, knowledge, and fortitude on my side. I was prepared emotionally with a positive attitude and the support of most of my family and friends. I was prepared physically because I used my knowledge about nutrition and the immune system to build up my body's strength and healing mechanisms.

I visualized how I would look and feel without my last little scarred-up breast. I visualized how much safer from a recurrence of breast cancer I would be in the future. All of this worked well for me. I can honestly say I haven't missed that breast anything close to the way I mourned the first one. It seems strange to say it, but I had already let go of my left breast before it was cut away from my body. Even so, there has been an adjustment to the scar and being so flat chested. Oh, I knew I would be flat chested, and even joked about it beforehand. I just didn't know how extreme it would be.

The one thing I forgot about the whole deal was the *pain!* I used everything I knew about healing, stress, and a positive attitude, along with the pain medication, to get me through the first weeks after surgery. I wasn't worried about whether I was doing well or not. I knew I was doing well enough to suit myself. Furthermore, I felt safer, and I was happy it was all over. I would never need to have another mastectomy!

In retrospect, if I had it all to do over from the beginning, knowing what I know now, there are some things I might have done differently. But I can't turn back the clock and I can't see into the future, so I am content with the knowledge that I made the best decisions for myself that I could at the time. I trust I will continue to do so in the future.

A Daughter's Viewpoint

When I found out that Mom had breast cancer, the first thing that went through my mind was that she was going to die. I didn't know anything about cancer except that you usually associate it with pain and death.

I cried a lot at first. I didn't know what to say or do and I was mad. I was mad because I knew that there were so many things that Mom wanted to do with her life, and she hadn't done them yet. My brother and I were just at the age where we were moving out of the house and then Mom was supposed to have all that time for herself. Then she found out that she had breast cancer.

It made me think a lot about my life. I quit smoking and I was determined to try to do what I wanted with my life *now* and not put it off, because we just don't know how much longer we will be here. You really should live for the day.

I had an eight month–old daughter and was thinking about having another baby when we found out that Mom had cancer. At first, I didn't even know if I should have another baby. It all seems silly now. I realized that life has to go on and we all just have to keep on living the best we can.

When Mom started her chemotherapy, I was lost. I wanted to help her, but I felt like I was more in the way when I tried to help. I think that if family members really want to help, they should seek advice and learn more about the right way to help someone with cancer who is going through chemotherapy. It isn't something that you automatically know about. You need to learn—and I wish that I could have had more time to devote to learning, for my mother's sake.

I felt for my mom because she had lost her breast (now both of them). Being a woman, I can't imagine how terrible that must feel. I worried about my mom and dad's relationship a little. Not too much, because I felt that my dad loved my mother more than anything in this world and he would always be there for her. I think that he might not have known what to do while she was going through everything, and as a result might not have been as supportive as she needed him to be.

My mother has a strong will to live and to fight whatever she comes up against. I have a good feeling about everything now. I feel that she is going to make the most of her life now. She still has problems with her arms and with her strength. She gets tired easily and I keep having to remind myself of these things.

As a result of my mother having had cancer, I have realized that life is very fragile and shouldn't be taken lightly. Tell your loved ones how much you love them every chance you get. It might be your last. Don't put off important things like these until tomorrow.

I'm really glad my mom goes to a support group.

She has learned a lot of interesting things and shares them with me and everyone else.

My attitude toward life now reminds me of one of my mom's favorite poems by Jenny Joseph:

Warning

When I am an old woman, I shall wear purple
With a red hat which doesn't go, and doesn't suit me.
And I shall spend my pension on brandy and summer gloves
And satin sandals, and say we've no money for butter.
I shall sit down on the pavement when I am tired
And gobble up samples in shops and press alarm bells
And run my stick along the public railings
And make up for the sobriety of my youth
I shall go out in my slippers in the rain
And pick the flowers in other people's gardens
And learn to spit.

But now we must have clothes that keep us dry
And pay our rent and not swear in the street
And set a good example for the children.
We will have friends to dinner and read the papers.

But maybe I ought to practice a little now?
So people who know me are not too shocked and surprised
When suddenly I am old and start to wear purple.

—*Jenny Joseph*

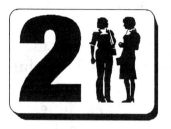 **ALLIE FAIR'S STORY**

It seems I had lived from one crisis to another most of my adult years. I had become so used to crises and deadlines that I felt almost lost if I wasn't putting out some kind of fire.

I was always trying to get everything in order, everything in place, and keep it that way. I always wanted to make everything just right for each person I cared about. My being a widowed parent of four children who had lost their father at an early age, I was always trying to compensate them for their loss. I wanted to give them all the love I could give, but I also wanted to give them the security of material things that other children received from their fathers, even if it meant working two or three jobs, eating lunch while driving or working, and sleeping only a few hours a night.

I was a perfectionist at everything I attempted. You have heard about "Type A" behavior. Well, think about "Type A Plus" behavior! My life was so stressful. I put all my energy into being a super mom or being the employee with the zero error rate and 100% accuracy. I was always there for someone else. I did not have enough hours in the 24 hours of the day to take care of myself.

I had a lot of anger, frustration, and resentment inside because I had lost my husband and the children had lost their father. We were continuously faced with financial difficulties, various illnesses and family problems. Is it any wonder that after fifteen years of stress that I was diagnosed with breast cancer?

It was Wednesday, November 15, 1989, at approximately 1:00 PM, that I received the telephone call telling me I had breast cancer. This call turned my world upside down. My mind filled with confusion and fear. I felt my life was shattered and my future so uncertain. I had never thought that I would have to undertake a battle against breast cancer.

That Wednesday, I was checking cases in my office at the Department of Social Services. I had decided to go to lunch later that day because I had so much work to get done. The office was very quiet, as most of my co-workers had gone to lunch already. There was an almost eerie silence in the air.

I walked down the quiet, vacant hall to put cases on a co-worker's desk. Although I was only gone for a couple of minutes, when I returned, I decided to check my voice mail. There was a message from my surgeon. I felt a little nervous, but I told myself he was calling to tell me that the growth he had removed the previous Friday was benign.

I dialed his telephone number and he answered on the first ring. He said, "I'm sorry to have to tell you on the telephone, but the growth was malignant." He told me to come to his office anytime that afternoon. The overwhelming impact of the surgeon's words made it impossible for me to hear anything else he said to me.

I became numb. I was so scared. *Cancer* is a very scary word. Only those people who have been told they have cancer can understand just how frightening this experience is. My first thought was, I have cancer. My mother died of cancer in 1982. Am I going to die of cancer? Dear God, I want to live. I'm only 52 years old and there is so much living I still want to do. Why me? My children lost their father. Are they going to lose their mother? I began to shake all over. After all, I had been one of those persons who had regular check-ups and yearly mammograms. Why me? Why now? Why? Why? *WHY*?

I called my supervisor. Within seconds, she was there with me. We called my daughter at her place of employment. Somehow I told her. She sounded so calm and said she was busy and could she call me back. In less than two minutes, she called back, very upset. Crying, she said she would meet me at the surgeon's office. Only the Friday before, she and I had gone Christmas shopping at the new mall, while my breast was still numb from the outpatient surgery. We had laughed about our shopping spree that day.

My office mate returned from lunch and insisted on driving me to the doctor's office, where my daughter was waiting for us in the parking lot. We hugged and cried, then went inside to talk with the surgeon. The surgeon seemed as shocked as we were. He had said all along that he was 98% sure it was just a benign cyst.

I probably talked and cried for almost two hours. He advised us there were tests and scans to do before scheduling surgery. He explained to us if the cancer had metastasized or spread to other areas, there would be no need to operate and remove the breast. He said the nurse would call to schedule a CAT scan and bone scan, and then would call me that afternoon to tell me when I was scheduled.

I asked my daughter to please drive me back to my office. I didn't feel that I could go home right then. I could not tell my sixteen–year old son that I had cancer. Later, I learned that my daughter had picked him up at school and told him, and also had called my daughter and son who were living in Winston-Salem.

So many friends at work came by my office that evening to give me a hug and to shed a tear with me. They reached out to give me love and support. I needed that support! I didn't realize just how much I needed that support until days later.

I called my church office and talked with my pastor, who said he would meet me at my home.

I had a telephone call from the surgeon's office

advising me that I was scheduled at 7:30 the following morning for the tests and scans.

Since the growth was malignant, I was suddenly
hurled into the world of nuclear medicine, x-rays,
operating rooms, endless tubes, drains, and needles—
plus the terror of the unknown, the exhaustion of
living in a rebellious body, the frustration of some
insensitive friends, but also the relief of finding
others who did truly care and understand.

My daughter and my pastor spent the following
day at the hospital with me. I was so frightened and
anxious while waiting to get the tests results. I did a
lot of praying. I guess I was really scared about the
bone scan, as I had already had so much bone and
joint pain for months. Upon completion of tests and
scans, my daughter and I went straight to the
surgeon's office. I did not want any telephone conversations with him.

We arrived there and expressed our concerns to
the lovely lady at the desk. My surgeon had not
returned from surgery at the hospital. Then the lady,
who much later I learned was the surgeon's wife,
said that normally she would not say anything, but
she knew how anxious my daughter and I were, so
she told us the hospital had just called and the scans
were negative.

My daughter and I began crying tears of joy.
About this time, the doctor arrived at the office. He
rejoiced with us, and then it was time to talk about
my choices and options. I would like to go back and

tell you a little about the months prior to this diagnosis. About two years earlier, I had been diagnosed with fibrocystic breast disease. My breast had hurt occasionally and also had a burning sensation. On a couple of occasions I had clear drainage from the breast and my internist had sent me for a mammogram. Many times when I had bone and joint pain, I also had pain in my right breast. I would rub Aspercreme over my breast, as well as on my arms and legs. I had been under the care of several doctors for the past seven years, having been treated for bone and joint pain, rheumatoid arthritis, high blood pressure, fibromyalgia, irritable colon syndrome, and also checked for lupus and connective tissue disease. I really did not need any more problems.

In June and July of 1989, I had been out of work due to excruciating pain in bones, joints, muscles, and my entire body. During this time, I had found a hard knot, about the size of a small June pea, near the surface of the skin on the underside of my right breast. It seemed to just appear overnight.

I was checked by my internist, who referred me to a surgeon that same day. The surgeon checked the knot and tried to do a needle aspiration, with no success. He told me he was still 98% sure it was a benign cyst, but if there was any change, to return to see him.

A few months later, in October, I noticed the knot had grown from the size of the small June pea to that of a "jolly green giant" pea. Every day for a week, I thought about calling the surgeon, but I kept hoping I would wake up one morning and the knot would have disappeared.

Finally, one night I had a very vivid dream. I dreamed that I had breast cancer and had to have surgery. Now I am convinced that God was telling me in a dream that I had breast cancer and to do something about it.

At this point, I would like to interject this advice to everyone: *"Be aware of your own feelings," "Take action,"* and *"Don't sit back while the doctor or surgeon waits."* I should have insisted that the knot be surgically removed five months earlier. I called the surgeon the following day, and told him about the rapid growth change in the lump. I was scheduled for a biopsy in his office a few days later.

On that day, I went to the surgeon's office where, under a local anesthetic, he removed the growth. He had to make two incisions, as it was attached in two places. The growth appeared jagged. It was white, with some yellow tinges and a few pink streaks. The pathology report gave the size as 1.2 x 0.8 x 0.6 cm, and the diagnosis was infiltrating ductal carcinoma.

Taking Charge

The days between my diagnosis and surgery were busy ones. I realized that I must learn everything I could about breast cancer—my options, my choices, and the treatments. I knew that I had to take charge and be in control. I knew that I must fight for my life harder than I had ever fought for anything.

I don't recall the exact order that I did things the next few weeks, however, I know that I did a lot. I spent hours searching through books, magazines, and newspapers. I read everything I could find on breast cancer.

Some of the material I read scared me, but that was better than not knowing. I felt much more in control once I understood my disease and what was happening to me. I called the Cancer Information Service's cancer "hot line" (which is listed under "Sources" at the end of this book), and any other numbers I felt could answer any of my questions.

I talked to physicians and medical personnel. I called a psychologist whom I knew had helped to form a therapy support group, called Life After Cancer–Pathways, a few years earlier. He met with me that evening at 7:00 PM, and advised me to go to the therapy support group the following morning (three days after my diagnosis).

I realized that if I had to deal with cancer, I had to be as positive as I could be. I was very determined to fight for my life. I did not plan to leave any stone unturned. So I made plans to go to the therapy support group the following morning. All during this time, I kept thinking that if there were one person in the world with whom I'd like to talk, it was Dr. Lewis Rathbun. He had been my OB-GYN doctor for almost 20 years before he retired.

I knew he had helped to start the Life After

Cancer therapy support group. I had no idea that he still worked with the group each Saturday, or that he would be the first person with whom I would talk at the meeting. He answered many questions for me. There were four of us at the orientation meeting that morning. The regular meeting was held after orientation.

At the therapy support group that first day, I met a lovely young woman, Donna, who was in her early thirties and was the mother of two small children. She told me that she had breast cancer and had a mastectomy about five months earlier. She had also had four months of chemotherapy. She recommended a book called *Choices,* written by Marion Morra and Eva Potts. This book traveled with me everywhere I went for the next few weeks.

I'll always remember how my new friend stood in the parking lot and talked with me for almost an hour after the meeting. She talked with me about her surgery and her treatments and answered a lot of my questions. She kept encouraging me and telling me that if she could do it, anyone could do it.

I really felt she was my "angel unaware," sent to talk with me. She continued to call me daily, speaking words of encouragement. She told me to be open and receptive to all the love and support my family and friends had to offer. She emphasized the importance of hugs and sharing things with each other. I learned so much that day.

My friends and co-workers from the office were

very supportive during this waiting period. I received a lot of support from staff, supervisors, and co-workers. They invited me to their Christmas luncheon, their Christmas party, and anything they felt would keep me busy or visiting the office.

I talked to other women who had breast cancer. They shared with me their feelings about their disease and their treatments. They offered me their support.

I had more medical checkups and a mammogram, which did not show any lumps. I continued to go for counseling on a one-on-one basis, as well as to the group therapy sessions. I had a lot of fears—not only about the cancer, but also about the surgery. I had a fear of "being put to sleep." I had moments of despair, fear and anxiety about everything.

Those days were so difficult. I did not like to go to sleep at night, for I knew when I awoke, my first thought would be "I have cancer." My worst times seemed to be the early morning hours. I would try to get out of bed just as soon as I woke up, so I would not think as much about cancer, pain, and the possibility of dying. I'm sure every woman ever diagnosed with breast cancer wonders and dreads what tomorrow could bring.

Surgery

Eventually, my surgery was scheduled for December 1, 1989. We had decided on a lumpectomy, even though I had accepted the fact that I might have a mastectomy. I was referred to a radiation oncologist, who took much time listening to and answering my questions. I had been advised that after a lumpectomy, I would need radiation.

Although I do not recall much about Thanksgiving that year, I do remember my family being there. My sister-in-law came to stay with me until after my surgery. My daughter put up our Christmas tree during the Thanksgiving holidays. We decorated the tree so we could enjoy it some before my surgery. Other than that, it was like a blackout. I don't remember anything else between Thanksgiving and November 30, the day I went into the hospital.

My children were having a difficult time dealing with my illness. Their father had died during open heart surgery on December 22, 1974. I think they associated my surgery scheduled for December with his dying on the operating table in December, 1974. They were so afraid of losing me. I was glad to have my sister-in-law (who had been like my other mother) with me and the children during this period of time. The time passed rather quickly between Thanksgiving and the time I entered the hospital.

I entered Memorial Mission Hospital on November 30, 1989, about 1:00 PM. My room was in 7 East, the cancer wing. The nurses were wonderful, and kept checking on me after I got settled in my room.

One of the nurses brought me surgery forms to sign. I noticed the form was for a mastectomy, but I signed it anyway. Later, my surgeon came by and told me I had been given the wrong form to sign. He said that he would have them bring me a form to sign for the lumpectomy, and that he would tear up the form for the mastectomy. I insisted on signing both forms, and told him that I wanted him to do whatever was necessary, even if it was a mastectomy. I wanted to get rid of all the cancer. I trusted my surgeon to do only what was necessary.

I think my intuition was guiding me. You see I'm one of those people who believes in listening to your body and to your feelings. As it turned out, my intuition was pretty good.

My surgery was scheduled for the next morning, Friday, at 8:00 AM. I couldn't sleep much that night, so I listened to a lot of cassettes, read, and prayed a lot. I took a sleeping pill and slept a few hours.

In those early morning hours, I awoke and could not return to sleep. I heard the sounds of the hospital awakening—the low murmurs of voices. Each sound signaled the moving of the clock hand closer to the hour of my surgery.

Finally, I got out of bed, showered, and washed my hair. I stood at the mirror and looked at my breasts. I tenderly held my breast in my hand, for I knew there was a possibility that when I awoke, my soft tender breast might no longer be a part of me. My knees began shaking. The tears again began to slide down my cheeks. I asked God to please give me the strength I needed for whatever I faced. I prayed for my family, and asked God to comfort each one.

A nurse came in to give me pre-operative sedation about 6:15 AM. I was to swallow three pills with one sip of water. It would take awhile to have the desired effect of calming me down—not enough time before the operation, yet I took the medication anyway. Once orders are written, I guess they are carried out, no matter what—but I recognized the medication I was given, and realized it would take much more to sedate me.

A few minutes later, my daughter arrived. Then my pastor arrived and said a beautiful prayer for me. My internist, who had spent so much time talking with me the past few weeks, came to my room. He went down to the pre-op room and waited with me until my surgeon's assistant arrived.

The pre-op room was cold. I was shivering. A very kind nurse came over to me and placed a warm, soft blanket over me. She tried to make me comfortable. I recognized the patient beside me. I spoke to her and we chatted briefly. I was awake, but felt a little more relaxed. For weeks, I had the fear of not waking up after my surgery. That fear was gone now. I felt very peaceful.

I had asked my surgeon if he would order medication so I would not remember the operating room. I remember the attendants starting to roll me toward the operating room. I saw the doors as we started through them. I remembered nothing more until I was in the recovery room and my surgeon came in to tell me that he had found more cancer and had to remove the breast.

I asked the nurse the time. She told me it was 10:20. (Three times after surgery and prior to this surgery, I had awakened at 10:20). I was in so much pain! I was having difficulty breathing, so I was receiving oxygen. The nurse kept checking my vital signs. I was so thankful to be alive and to have awakened from the anesthesia.

As the sedation wore off, I was aware of excruciating pain. The nurse continued to give me pain medication. Shortly, I was told we would be returning to my room. I was anxious to get out of the recovery room, for all around me I could hear moans and groans of others trying to handle their own postoperative pain.

It seemed only a few minutes until I was on my way back to my room. I was wide awake and fully alert. I had my own "cheering section" in the hall outside my room. There was my beautiful daughter, her mother-in-law, my devoted sister-in-law, my sister, and my two supervisors. I spoke and called each one by name.

Soon, I was in bed in my room. The room seemed to be moving. I remember trying to talk, but my mouth was too dry. I was in pain again, and I was given morphine, the self–administered type. I could just press a button and get a pre-measured amount every few minutes. I slept very little the rest of the afternoon. However, I vaguely remember some friends stopping by during the evening.

My surgeon came by later in the evening and explained to me that he had found a large cancer embedded back of the nipple area in the right breast. Later, the surgeon's assistant came by to see me. He told me there was no choice but to remove the breast because of the size of the cancer found during the operation.

A former co-worker stayed with me the night of my surgery. My supervisor came and stayed for several hours. I felt the love and support they offered and it meant so very much to me. The following day, my surgeon came to my room smiling. He said he had removed sixteen lymph nodes—all were negative. This pleased us very much. However, since the cancer was 6.0 x 4.0 cm and had spread to the surrounding breast tissue and skin, he said he had called in an oncologist to discuss chemotherapy.

I don't remember much about the weekend, but I was scared on Monday after talking with the oncologist who recommended chemotherapy. That week I had to have a MUG scan of the heart and more tests, as one of the chemotherapy drugs was to be adriamycin.

The Best Christmas Ever

I was hospitalized for ten days. On a Sunday, I was discharged. I was very anxious to go home—to my room. I admit I had a lot of anxiety about going home, because I would not have the nurses coming into my hospital room reassuring me I was doing fine. Upon arriving home, my family had tried to have everything nice for me—good food, lovely flowers—and friends from my church dropped by to visit.

I was not able to drive for three weeks. The day after arriving home from the hospital, I had to call my surgeon, who began aspirating fluid from under my arm every other day. Christmas was only a few days away. I was so glad I had done most of my Christmas shopping early. Also, I had been a representative for Avon and for the House of Lloyd products, so I had a closet full of gifts from which I could shop. I found that I was very slow in wrapping gifts. I tired very easily. My son's girlfriend came over and helped me do gift wrapping.

The Christmas tree was so beautiful that year. My daughter had put up the tree and decorated it for me during Thanksgiving. I recalled so many times in the past when we all got mad because lights weren't working, the tree didn't look straight, or for some other reason. But not this time—the tree symbolized the tree of life; the lights reminded me of Jesus, the Light of the world; the gifts symbolized God's Gift, His Son.

On Christmas Day, all my children were home for the first time in several years. My dad, stepmother, sister, and her family came for the day. I wondered if all my family came home because they expected me to die before another Christmas. A few times, I had to go to my room to cry. However, I think this was the best Christmas Day in many, many, many years.

All too soon, it was over. My family returned to their homes, except for my sister-in-law, who was to be my caretaker during my chemotherapy treatments. I don't remember much about the next few days. I do remember that one of my best friends came up from Charleston to spend a few days and a friend from Winston-Salem came and spent some time with me during the New Year holidays. On January 3, 1990, I was to go for my third chemotherapy treatment.

Chemotherapy

A real trauma of my cancer experience was chemotherapy, which began on December 20, 1989.

I wanted to wait until after the holidays to start my chemotherapy, however, my oncologist told me that I was at high risk for a recurrence and that he didn't want me to wait. He said my cancer had probably been growing for five to seven years, because of the size of the cancer. He said that one of the first signs of breast cancer was sometimes bone and joint pain. He explained to me that it was possible that the breast cancer was in a growing spurt whenever I was in so much pain, and that when the cancer was lying dormant, the bone and joint pain subsided.

My first treatment was on a cold day with lots of snow flurries. I was scheduled to have a treatment every Wednesday at 11:00 AM for the next six months. I became very anxious wondering "what if" it snowed so much that I had to miss an appointment.

For the first treatment, I carried my cassette player and a relaxation tape with me. Although I was scared, I wanted to appear confident. I wanted to act and look as if I was in control, although I must admit at that point, I did not feel in control.

The nurse weighed and measured me so that the oncologist could compute my body surface area and prescribe the dosage of Cytoxan, adriamycin, and fluorouracil for the outlined protocol (CAF). I would receive my chemo intravenously. Before the treatment, I would be given Phenergan, Ativan, Reglan, and Benadryl for the nausea and side effects.

During the first treatment, I fell asleep almost immediately. Later, after the chemo drip had stopped, my oncologist woke me up. I don't remember much about leaving the office or the trip home. My daughter would drive me to and from the big treatments— which was every fourth treatment. My sister in law was there to care for me when I arrived home. My children who lived out of town would call.

Later, I learned that I would always talk to them, but I would not remember talking to them. These treatments were the most devastating experiences, medically and emotionally, that I have ever had. I felt I was actually on a journey through hell. There was such a dread of entering the oncology building. Waiting for the reactions, which varied in severity from treatment to treatment, was excruciating.

After every chemotherapy treatment, I was violently ill. The antinausea drugs did not seem to be that effective for me. However, I do realize that today's medications are for people like me. I'm so thankful we have them, although there were times when I felt I would die from the treatments.

So many times, I considered quitting chemotherapy. It drained me to the point it seemed I was only existing. It seemed my whole life was planned around chemotherapy treatments. However, I have wondered just how much worse I would have been without them.

I felt so out of control during this period of time—I was unable to deal with my own life, not to speak of trying to help my teenage son, who was having great difficulty coping with my disease and my treatments. Although I tried to keep "hanging in there," I had so much fear and anxiety. After some of the treatments on Wednesdays, I would feel well enough for someone to drive me to my therapy support group on Saturdays. After the big treatments, it would be Monday or Tuesday before I felt like going outside again.

It seemed I began having major side effects in early February. I really thought I was going to die. Sometimes, I was so sick that I would lie in the bathroom floor rather than try to go back to bed in my room. My mouth and esophagus had sores, for which I was prescribed a mouthwash known as "Miracle Mouthwash." I must say, it really did work! It helped tremendously.

My eyes became inflamed, almost like a burn from

a sunlamp. I was given a prescription for a small bottle of eye drops which cost $25, however, they did relieve my eyes. My lungs felt scorched. I had so much difficulty breathing and my chest was heavy. My heart skipped beats, and at times it felt as if my heart would jump out of my chest. I would have hot flashes, then cold chills. At times, I would have cold sweats. My head hurt. My hair was falling out. Sometimes, my head felt so hot it seemed I could hear my hair crackling. I would raise up in bed and look at my pillow to see if my thinning hair was all out and on the pillow. Whenever I bathed, I would see lots of hair floating on the water. This made me so sad. Tears would drip down my face, neck, and chest until I thought I could hear them hitting the bath water.

As if hair loss, mouth sores, nausea, vomiting, diarrhea, and pain were not enough, I could not remember things. I was so forgetful. I would start to tell someone something, and I would completely forget what I was talking about. This was scary, because I would begin wondering if the cancer had spread to my brain.

At times, I would have hallucinations, thinking I saw things that were not there. One night, I was trying to watch a television program with my sister-in-law. I kept thinking I saw a large rat about a foot tall sitting between me and the television. I began crying. My sister-in-law came to comfort me. She kept reassuring me that I was OK. Without her support and tender loving care, I do not know what might have happened to me. She was the only person who saw me during my worst moments. She saw my struggle to survive.

Oftentimes, any loud noise frightened me. Sometimes, just the sound of the telephone ringing would scare me. I was so insecure and afraid. I was even more frightened if any of my family went away. In February, my daughter and her husband went on a week's vacation. I was afraid that I would die while they were out of town.

On March 4, I went for a chemotherapy treatment. After my lab work and examination, my oncologist informed me that we were stopping the treatments due to the problems I was having with the adriamycin.

As much as I disliked having chemo, I was disappointed, discouraged, and frightened when the doctor stopped the treatments. If I couldn't tolerate the chemo—then what about fighting cancer? The chemo had represented a type of security for me, even with the adverse side effects. To have this security blanket yanked away made me feel like I was standing naked in zero temperature.

I arrived home and told my son that my treatments had stopped. We both became upset and angry. We were yelling and throwing things—everything from a cassette player to a skateboard. My son was telling me "You can't stop the treatments" and "I don't want you to die." He kept yelling that it was not his fault that I had cancer and that he was sorry.

After awhile, we both calmed down, cried, and began talking. I think this was the first time I realized that my son was blaming himself for my cancer. I tried to reassure him that I would continue to fight for my life.

I was thankful that my oncologist had cautiously monitored my care and tried to help alleviate any problems. I was also thankful to have had the few months of chemotherapy treatments, which may have killed any cancer cells left. I recently read an article that said that new studies have found that the CAF protocol of chemo may be as effective when given for four months as other chemotherapy drugs that are given for six months.

Also, I decided that I would just have to do my relaxation, my visual imagery, and make my T-Cells go on a "search and destroy" mission to kill any unwanted cells.

The day chemotherapy stopped, I was sent to my surgeon. He was to schedule me within three weeks for another surgery to revise the mastectomy scar and remove excess tissue that the body had not absorbed. I was also advised that I would be taking radiation treatments as soon as I was recovered from the surgery. I felt that I had "hit a brick wall" again.

The pain inside was more from feeling *alone* than from the impending surgery and radiation. My children were angry about further surgery and treatments. They began to withdraw from me, maybe detaching themselves due to fear. My surgery was

April 5. I spent seven days in the hospital. I had lots of tests before I could have the surgery, but I did fine. Three weeks later, I began radiation treatments.

My Radiation Experience

I had met a radiation oncologist when I thought I was going to have a lumpectomy. After my modified radical mastectomy and while undergoing chemotherapy, I learned that I would need to have 25 radiation treatments because my breast cancer was also in the skin and surrounding breast tissue.

Radiation treatments consist of using x-rays at high levels to destroy the ability of cells to grow and divide. Both normal cells and diseased cells are affected, but most normal cells are able to recover quickly.

In my case, radiation was used as an adjuvant treatment, in addition to surgery, chemotherapy, and the hormonal therapy with tamoxifen, which had begun when my chemo stopped.

The machine used for my radiation treatment was the *linear accelerator.* This is the "big gun" of cancer treatment. This machine delivers two types of radiation at different energy levels. It produces electromagnetic waves. When it is turned on, it changes electricity into high energy beams. Very complex calculations are needed to determine the dosage and timing of treatments.

My radiation team consisted of several people in addition to the radiation oncologist. There were radiation physicists who planned the treatments designed to deliver the desired doses of radiation, and kept the linear accelerator working properly. There was also a nurse, a radiation therapy technologist, and radiation technicians.

I went alone to my first appointment with the radiation oncologist. As I stated earlier, I had already met him soon after my diagnosis. He had also spoken at my breast cancer support group meeting one evening. I had immediately liked him. He discussed every detail of my medical history and also talked to my internist and my rheumatologist. He took so much time explaining the treatments to me. He agreed with my oncologist and surgeon about the treatment plan. He explained to me the areas he would radiate including the collar bone area and the chest area. He told me that a major side effect of radiation would be fatigue.

Before I could actually start radiation therapy, I had to go through a couple of hours of what they call *simulation*, a procedure in which they find the exact location they want to radiate. Very complex calculations are needed to determine the dosage and timing of treatments. After the simulation process, I had red and black markings drawn on my chest to outline the boundaries. This sure was a reminder of my status as a cancer patient. It was almost like having the "scarlet letter" painted on, except in this case, the letter was "C."

I was anxious to get on with these treatments. I

had so many frequent doctor appointments that I had little time left over for doing anything else. I was spending a lot of time and energy protecting my life.

I was scheduled for the 25–day radiation protocol. Each day, I would arrive at the hospital and go to Radiation Therapy. I would register with the receptionist, walk through a hall, put on the hard–to–manage backless gown, and sit quietly in the "gown" waiting room with other patients, waiting to hear my name called.

Although there was a physical closeness, there was sometimes emotional isolation. People stared straight ahead. Some patients stared into space. Some patients held onto a family member's arm, while others slumped in wheel chairs. Of course, some patients were sicker than others. Occasionally, I talked with someone. Oftentimes, I read or just sat quietly. I learned that there were patients from all over Western North Carolina who had traveled two hours to get to radiation therapy and would have to travel two hours to return home. On Fridays, the chaplain, David, came by to talk and to visit. He was an inspiration to me.

I thought radiation would be a breeze, since I had had it so rough in chemo. However, with the third treatment, I began to feel nauseated and have some of the same side effects that I had experienced with chemotherapy. I finally learned that this sometimes happens. It is known as *chemo recall*. I was given medication for the nausea and advised to rest a lot because of my extreme fatigue. One must remember that everybody's symptoms are different. Not everyone has such adverse side effects.

When my name was called, I walked to the radiation room where the technicians conversed. I stepped up on a stool, lay down on the table and removed my gown from the right shoulder. Over me hung the huge machine. The right half of my chest was bared. Together, the technicians aligned the light from the machine with the markings on my chest area. The technician stretched out my right arm and asked me to grasp a handle to keep my arm steady. My tender chest and incision hurt from the extended position.

The room lights were dimmed so that the treatment set–up could be guided by the light from the linear accelerator. The table was raised and lowered—to the right, to the left. The technician would mark or re-mark on spots as the doctor directed. I was advised not to wash off the marks. The technician would leave the room. Through the intercom, I'd hear the instructions "Don't move." Then *whir-click, whir-click* sounded the machine. Sometimes, I counted. Oftentimes, I would say affirmations or comforting Bible verses or do visual imagery. Then the linear accelerator switched off.

A few treatments had to be postponed due to the appearance of burns on my neck and chest. Later, toward the end of my treatments, my skin turned red and became irritated. The rays seemed to go through my chest and had a sunburn effect on my back. There was a block of skin that turned very brown and remains brown two years later. My lungs and esophagus bothered me. I had some difficulty swallowing. I was unable to wear a bra or my prostheses. I had to wear soft, loose tops. The day after my 25th treatment, my skin became very irritated, dry, itchy, and oozing. Within the next two days, I had blisters and burns about the size of a half dollar.

My radiation oncologist saw me once a week during my treatments. After my treatments, he had to see me every other day for approximately three weeks due to my radiation burns, then twice a week for several weeks. Finally, I was able to wear a bra and my prosthesis. Another milestone accomplished!

About three weeks after my radiation stopped I fell and broke my foot. So my leg was in a cast to my knee. Two weeks after breaking my foot, I began having chest pains and difficulty breathing. One of my friends drove me to the emergency room, where I learned I had developed numerous blood clots in both lungs. I was once again hospitalized. I was in the hospital for twelve days.

During this period of time, I became very depressed. I wondered why I wanted to live. It seemed that I had nothing to look forward to. I felt doomed. I thought tomorrow will only be a continuation of today and today is as painful as yesterday. The chaplain spent several hours with me that day. A psychiatrist was called in to talk with me. The mental anguish and the emotional torment were as painful as the physical aspects of my life.

When I returned home, I continued going for counseling on a one-to-one basis as well as to the therapy support group. I was a fighter those next few months! Although I was in constant pain, I dragged myself up to go with my son for some counseling sessions. Less than three months later, I had to resign from my job of twelve years, as my doctors advised me that I was unable to return to work due to my multiple health problems.

There came a time when I was at home alone for three months. During this time, I did a lot of praying, listening to relaxation tapes, and visual imagery. It was once again the holiday season. I decorated my Christmas tree—even though I was alone until Christmas Eve. The tree was once again so beautiful. Many nights, as I sat alone I would watch the flashing lights and the twinkling star and reminisce of days long gone by. Again, I knew I wanted to live!

It seemed I had fair sailing for a few months. Then in March, 1991, I went for a routine check-up. The following day, I received a telephone call from my oncologist's nurse. My liver function tests were extremely elevated. This meant a CAT scan, a bone scan, and another CAT scan a few months later. The scans were negative. Each month, I had more lab work. Once you have had breast cancer, it doesn't matter how many years you have survived, the fear of recurrence is always with you.

After much research, telephone calls, and doctor

visits, I made the decision to stop my hormonal therapy drug, tamoxifen, for a period of time. I was having a lot of problems, such as difficulty breathing, nausea, and fatigue, which I felt might be related to the medication. I discussed this decision with my oncologist, and he agreed with me—if this was what I wanted to do. It appeared that I might be in the three to five percent of women who have adverse side effects to tamoxifen. Although it helped lower my cholesterol, it might have caused me some life threatening problems such as blood clots. I would get so short of breath after walking up just a few steps. I was using oxygen at night, as my oxygen level dropped into a danger zone whenever I slept. Later, I learned that the oxygen problem was a sleep disorder related to my having fibromyalgia, and not actually from the tamoxifen.

After my liver function tests were back in the normal zone, I decided once again to talk with my doctors about resuming the tamoxifen. My doctors all agreed that this was a good idea, but that I would have to continue to take the anticoagulant (Coumadin) while I was taking the tamoxifen. Also, we decided that I would have lab work each month for several months.

My Lessons

After the surgeries and treatments for breast cancer, it has been somewhat difficult for me to get back to a well world. There is always some fear and anxiety. The care and support you receive during treatments give you a sense of security. The road to recovery can have many potholes. Too many people do not realize that the psychological consequences of cancer are as devastating as the physical ones.

I continue to have frequent check-ups. Sometimes, I get tired of going for appointments, and long to be free from nurses, needles, and nausea, but even that relief would be tempered with unexpected insecurity. There will always be a risk of getting breast cancer again. I worry about a recurrence. Every illness carries some fear. However, I have learned that for me, one of my best coping techniques is being in the PsychoSocial Therapy Support Group and the breast cancer support group. My counselors have helped me learn to live in the moment. I have met some very dear friends in the support groups.

I have learned to feel the love of so many people. I have learned to deal with feelings of resentment, anger, guilt, and criticism. I no longer blame others, but rather take responsibility for my own experiences. I have learned to be more gentle and kind to myself. I have learned to forgive myself and to love myself unconditionally.

I am not a different woman because of breast cancer. I am a changed woman. Having breast cancer changed me in many ways—not just physically, but emotionally and spiritually. It taught me tough lessons about loyalty and love. My priorities have changed. I began to listen to my inner self. Having breast cancer also taught me that life cannot be predicted. Some effort had to be made to wake up and live each day as if it mattered. I am more confident now. I care less about what others think and I do what I think is right for me. I have choices. Also, I take more risks now. I find that the risks I take bring more fullness to my life than I have known before.

I have "let go" of a lot of garbage and old, self defeating messages. I can see myself through eyes of love. I have found new strengths and new meanings—now I am taking care of me! I feel more in control of my life. Faith, hope, and the will to live are so important to me. I feel I am living from day to day here on earth. My attitude has changed. Although I have some long–term goals, I realize that life is always short and you can't put it on hold—you can only *go for it*.

I am not perfect. I don't even try to be perfect, but I am enjoying some quality moments. There are still so many things I would like to do, and so many places I would like to go. I love life and living. I am striving for some good quality time. I enjoy my calligraphy class. I would like to try an art class.

There is just so much beauty in this world. I see beauty in each day. I don't have moments to waste on "I should haves" and "what ifs." I take time to stop and smell the flowers—the golden daffodils, the lovely cherry blossoms, the pink and white dogwoods. I take time to admire the flaming, fiery azaleas, to view the dew on the rose petals, to catch a glimpse of a rainbow, and to enjoy the glowing sunrises and golden sunsets. I enjoy the sunshine, the raindrops, and the soft–falling white snow. I like to hear the bluebirds singing and the robins chirping. I like to watch the dancing butterflies. I no longer take such things for granted.

There are times I like the quietness of the evening. In the inner silence, I can create calm harmony and contentment. There is peace and serenity. Other times, I like the excitement of a circus and clowns. These are my moments. I must continue to make my time count. I like to give support to those I can help, just as I was given support by others. I am thankful that I had a second chance to enjoy "moments."

I have found that I have values and priorities that I did not realize. Through the knowledge that I have gained, I hope to benefit others. I want to be an inspiration to other women who have been diagnosed with breast cancer. I feel that each one of us is unique in our own way and need only follow our own star. I hope that by sharing my own personal story, I can make my time count. Each precious moment must count!

Angie's Story

It was late afternoon on a Wednesday in November, 1989. I came home from school to a very silent house. I knew that my aunt and my brother should be there.

I called out, as usual, "Anybody home?" Then I

looked in my aunt's room, and from the look on her face, I knew something was wrong.

When she told me that my sister had called to tell us that Mama had breast cancer, I think I completely went to pieces. I was so mad! How could happen to my mother who had been through so much already? It just wasn't fair. I thought back to the time Daddy died during surgery when we were little children. I was afraid Mama would die, too, and I couldn't do anything to help her. I remembered when Grandma died with cancer, and this scared me more.

I stalked around the house fussing, crying, and throwing things. Why? Why? Why?

When I became quiet, I found my brother in his room. He was not crying; he was staring into space as if dazed. I think he couldn't believe it either. Finally, he got himself under control enough to call, and we both talked with Mama. She told us that she would be all right and not to worry. Then my tears started and I cried for hours.

I'm thankful that Mama came through that surgery and the other things she has had to endure since then. I guess up until then, I took for granted that Mama would always be there—just as she had been for us during all those years she was raising us. I have realized since then that life cannot be taken for granted. Even though I cannot see my mother often since my work is in another city, I have tried to keep in touch often by telephone and to let her know that I love and appreciate her.

Chuck's Story

I had just gotten home from work that nice autumn evening, when the telephone rang. I didn't pay any attention, since for my aunt to talk to her friends was a usual thing.

A little later, I went by her room and noticed that she was crying. Then she told me about the phone call. My sister, who lives in the same town as my mom, had just called to tell us that Mom had found out she had breast cancer. She was already set up for all sorts of tests and scans by the time we heard.

It's hard for me to describe how I felt, but those words simply "knocked me for a loop." I couldn't believe it. My mom had been as both parents to me since I was a little boy and my dad had died. And now I might lose her, too! I felt that I could not bear it. For awhile, I was stunned. I couldn't talk to anyone. I was so scared that Mom would die or hurt and suffer a lot.

Finally, my aunt, sister, and I hugged each other and cried together. We began talking about when we could go up to see Mom. The telephone lines were kept rather busy during the next several weeks.

That was just before Christmas. We decided that all of us would go home and spend Christmas together. It felt so good to see Mom at home for Christmas.

I just want my Mom to know that I love her and will stay in touch as long as I live and will see her as often as I can.

Errata

Omission: Dedication page should read "To Dr. Lewis Rathbun with admiration and appreciation."

P. 14 Spelling: "*endemocarcinoma*" should read "adenocarcinoma."

P. 16 Spelling: "*wretched*" should read "retched."

P. 81-82 "*The support group leaders have taught me how to kindness. . .*" should read "The support group leaders have taught me how to improve the quality of my life with laughter and with kindness. . ."

P. 82 "*I'll always be grateful for the better I made in my life. . .*" should read "I'll always be grateful for the changes for the better I made in my life. . ."

P. 104, 109, 110, and 113 Spelling: "*dont's*" should read "don'ts."

P. 124 Spelling: "*Lymphopress*" should read "Lymphapress."

P. 149-150 "*Probably what sustains breast cancer patients with their treatments is the notion that their current how bad they feel. . .*" should read "Probably what sustains breast cancer patients with their treatments is the notion that their current discomfort often means longer survival—for no matter how bad they feel. . ."

Karen's Story

When I heard the word *cancer*, I felt like someone had knocked the breath out of me. My face felt clammy as the blood drained away and the panic rose up into my throat. My mother was going to die. In my mind, it was one and the same: *cancer* equals *death*.

It couldn't happen, not to my mother. Why, wasn't she invincible?! Nothing had ever broken her. She was the strongest person I had ever known. A super hero, able to leap tall buildings in a single bound. That was my mother. Any obstacle life had thrown at her, she had always handled and come out on top. Even as old as I was, this was how I saw her. She wasn't a mere mortal, made of flesh and blood. She was *my mother*.

I think that is why I had such a hard time dealing with everything—the chemotherapy, the radiation, the nausea, the need to lean on someone else. I had always looked at her with the eyes of a child. Now, I was having to grow up *fast*. My mind rejected all of this and, in doing so, my mother was the one to suffer. She needed my support and needed to feel loved. I tried to be there for her, but I let her down. I know that and I am sorry for it.

Oh, I listened to her when she needed to talk, I tried to help her with my brother, and I ran errands for her when she needed it, but emotionally there was a wall. She could feel it, I could feel it, and there was nothing that I seemed to be able to do to get past it. When she reached out to me, I backed away. She had to go elsewhere for the emotional support that she needed. She became involved with a cancer support group. I am extremely thankful to the friends she has made there. They know what she is going through and how to help her more than I could. When one of them says, "I know how you feel," it isn't just empty words of consolation. They really know how she feels. The love and friendship the support group has given her has eased some of the pressure off of me, and I have been able to come to terms with everything else.

It has been about three years since my mother was diagnosed with breast cancer. I am able to be more like the daughter I feel I should have been from the very beginning. I still feel rather inadequate because I am really just standing on the sidelines. I don't have the ability to fix everything and make it all right, but I can be there with a hug and a smile or a hand to hold when she needs it.

She is still the strongest person I have ever known. I look up to and admire her, not because I see her as an invincible superhero any longer, but because I accept her as she is, a mere mortal, made of flesh and blood. *My mother!*

Chris' Story

My mom getting cancer turned my world upside down. At first I thought, "No, this is not true—not my mom." She had always been so strong. She had kept the family together. Why would she get cancer?

A little later, I began wondering why she would hurt me by getting cancer. Did she no longer love me? She had always been a strict mom. As I was growing up, I often got angry with her because she was strict. There were times when I wished she would just go away, but I never wanted her to get cancer. I began to feel that it was my fault that mom had breast cancer. I felt that I was a disappointment to her and that she was "getting even" with me by getting cancer and maybe dying. I was scared to death.

I wanted our old life back. I wanted things to be normal again with us doing things as we had in the past—like mom going to work each day and picking me up at school in the evenings. I did not like to see her in pain, nor to hear her crying.

I was angry with everyone—myself, my family, and my mom. I was angry with God. My memories of my dad, if there were any at all, were so vague. If my mom died, what would happen to me? She was all I had left. I considered running away to avoid feeling the pain. I tried to heal my pain and escape the suffering by staying away from home as much as I could. Sometimes I walked, alone, for miles and miles.

I went to the beach with a friend and her family, where I tried to forget about mom's cancer, but there were times I wished the ocean waves would carry me far away.

Mom was participating in a cancer support group. There was a group for teenagers who had a family member with cancer. I began to attend the meetings and sometimes went with mom to her group. The counselors were so kind and caring. They seemed to understand my feelings, too. They didn't think I was bad or that I had caused mom to get cancer. They helped me to stop blaming myself and to see that there were things I could do which would help both my mom and me.

While the idea that mom could die still makes me lonely and afraid, I have grown up a lot. I have assumed more responsibility and I am not as insecure as I was. I am proud of myself for sticking around and trying to help. I realize now that I should give the ones I have all the love and care I can while they are living, so that if I do lose them, I will know I have done my best. I am thankful that I still have my mom!

I'd Pick More Daisies

If I had my life to live over again
I'd try to make more mistakes next time.
I would relax. I would limber up. I
Would be sillier than I have been this
Trip. I know of a very few things I
Would take seriously. I would take more

Trips. I would climb
more mountains,
Swim more rivers, and
watch more sunsets.
I would do more
walking and looking.
I would eat more ice
cream and less beans.
I would have more
actual troubles and

fewer imaginary ones. You see, I am one of those
People who live prophylactically and
Sensibly and sanely hour after hour,
Day after day. Oh, I've had my moments
And if I had it to do over again, I'd
Have more of them. In fact, I'd try to
Have nothing else. Just moments, one
After another, instead of living so many
Years ahead each day. I have been one of
Those people who never go anywhere without
A thermometer, a hot water bottle, a gargle,
A raincoat, aspirin, and a parachute.
If I had it to do over again,
I would go places, do things, and travel

Lighter than I have.
If I had my life to live over, I would
Start barefooted earlier in the spring
And stay that way later in the fall.
I would play hookey more. I wouldn't make
Such good grades except by accident.
I would ride on more merry-go-rounds.
I'd pick more daisies!

—Unknown

SUPPORT GROUPS

Life After Cancer-Pathways

Life After Cancer-Pathways is a therapy support group founded in April, 1977 by Lewis S. Rathbun, M.D., gynecological surgeon, and Donald R. Boone, M.S.W., A.C.S.W. Its purpose was to encourage cancer patients and their loved ones to fight for recovery.

Life After Cancer-Pathways offers a positive and practical approach to the emotional side of cancer. Patients are encouraged to become active participants in their recovery process by using all available resources—their emotions, hope, love, determination, purpose, and will to live.

Life After Cancer–Pathways encourages patients to learn all they can about their disease and its treatments in order to make informed choices. It offers educational services, has an extensive library with books, videos, and cassettes available for use by participants. It offers support services by having several support group meetings weekly from which patients and their families can choose to attend. It offers special groups for children and youth with cancer, and also for those who have family members with cancer. It offers special groups for spouses of those with cancer.

There are special services involving music, art, and play therapy. Intensive work within small groups in retreat settings is available.

The Life After Cancer-Pathways therapy support program offers both group and one-on-one counseling sessions to cancer patients, their families, and friends. The counselors and professionals with the therapy support group have a total of over 45 years experience in working with cancer patients and their families. They help these participants achieve a higher quality of life and enhance the possibility for recovery.

Techniques used include visual imagery, meditation, relaxation, working with inner wisdom, and goal setting. There are educational and informational programs, talks, and panels on a variety of wellness topics. Consultation and development services are available from highly trained volunteers.

Life After Cancer-Pathways does not charge for services. There is something for everyone from the point of diagnosis through long term survivorship. It is in support of, and in addition to, conventional medical treatment. It offers support in the hospital, in the home, or even by telephone. Life After Cancer-Pathways offers and provides services to participants to help them along their healing journey to recovery.

There are many such groups, in cities across the United States, which are available to help people with their fight to overcome cancer.

Allie Fair: My Support Group

Cancer touches nearly everyone's life, either directly or indirectly. It's vital, then, to understand how to live with the big "C."

Cancer is not just one disease. It is a group of more than two hundred diseases caused by abnormal cells that grow and can spread. While the search for cures and better treatments for all cancers continue, patients and their families and friends struggle with the physical, psychological, and financial hardship of the disease.

Cancer support groups meet a special need at a special time in life. They are intended to work with medical treatment, not to replace it. People say support groups help make a difference in their attitude towards life and the disease. Support groups offer more hope and less fear. They help people to better understand their disease as well as their treatments. They encourage family participation; and also offer a person without a family the opportunity to express himself or herself and to be accepted.

I found that one of the best things about a support group was realizing that I was not alone.

In a support group, you make friends. You find

them offering emotional support to help you through the bad times and rejoicing with you in the good times.

Research has shown that cancer patients and their families benefit from support groups. Besides reducing a woman's anxiety, support groups may also prolong her life. In a 1989 study in the British medical journal, *The Lancet*, David Spiegel, M.D., at the Stanford University School of Medicine in California, found that patients with metastatic breast cancer who attended weekly support groups lived eighteen months longer than those without such support.

Separate support groups for family members can help them air their fears and learn how to provide care for a loved one. A patient's family often goes through the same stages of emotions as the patient. However, they don't always go through the same stages at the same time. The patient may want to talk about her disease, but the family may still be in the denial phase and not want to talk about it. It is often hard for patients to talk to their families because they feel they will depress them. Thus, a support group for family members can be beneficial.

However, support groups may not be for everyone. There are some people who become depressed and don't want to deal with other patients' feelings. The key is to respect the way a woman chooses to cope with her illness, whether privately or openly.

Cancer does create a tremendous amount of fear—

the fear of death, the fear of pain and suffering. It gives you the feeling of being out of control. In a support group, patients learn how to live with their fears and to take more control of their lives. They learn how to participate in their treatment and how to talk to their doctor.

Someone has said the treatment of cancer can be just as devastating as the disease itself. The chemotherapy and radiation can cause patients to lose their hair and have nausea, fatigue, and insomnia. It's a feeling that your body is not the body you always lived in. You become very dependent on your doctor and on your family. It's a real sense of helplessness. Through a support group, you will get the benefit of moral support from other members of the group. Families and friends are wonderful, but they haven't been through that unique experience of being a cancer patient.

In my therapy support group, Life After Cancer–Pathways, I met so many lovely, precious people. There is a special bond because each of us experiences some of the same fears, anxieties, and problems. Each of us is dealing with the specter of death, as well as the struggle to live.

I personally met some very precious friends who were battling breast cancer. We talked about our disease, diagnosis, pathology reports, compared treatments, doctors, even compared scars, incisions, and prostheses. Each of us knew and understood how the others felt when they looked in the mirror at their bodies. We cried together, played games together, played bingo together, went to movies together, visited each other, and were always there for each other. We knew we could call each other any hour of the day or night if we had a problem we couldn't handle alone. We drove each other for tests, scans, and medical appointments. We had so much love to give each other.

Each of us had to make decisions about the disfigurement of our body, whether or not to have reconstructive surgery, the invasion of toxic chemicals into our bodies, and other choices. Some of us had financial difficulties, some had no insurance coverage, while others had constant struggles with insurance companies. Some of us had problems with our children at home as family dynamics shifted dramatically, some were coping with separations and divorces. Old priorities seemed to vanish in the space of a telephone call.

In breast cancer support groups, we shared everything, the most gut-wrenching of emotions. We told each other things we had never shared or told anyone else.

Each person will tell you that having breast cancer changes you in many ways, not just physically, but emotionally, and spiritually. It teaches you tough lessons about loyalty and love. You want to make amends in relationships. Your priorities change and your friends change. You begin to listen to your inner self—and you try to find out what you really want to do with your life. You learn to deal with your feelings of resentment, anger, and self hatred, and the feelings of guilt and criticism. You learn not to blame others, but rather to take responsibility for your own experiences.

What support we give out, we get back. We seek and receive support when we need support. We love and give support when others need our support. It is in our giving that we receive our healing.

I have changed in so many ways. Breast cancer forced me to confront emotionally all the elements of being a woman. Whatever may have been coming up before I had breast cancer, revealed itself after I had this disease. I no longer harbor feelings of resentment, guilt, or criticism. I have developed new priorities and values in my life.

Because of the therapy support group, I have learned to be more self confident. I have given myself permission to express my feelings of anger, fear, and anxiety. Through my therapy support group, I have learned to feel more at peace. I have found new strength and new meaning in my life, which I need in order to continue a life of fulfillment and true happiness. Sharing this information is one of the reasons I decided to co-author this book.

Lynne's Story

Lynne is one of the women we came in contact with through our therapy support group. In 1990, Lynne, an attractive redhead, was diagnosed with stage one breast cancer—intraductal carcinoma. She was 49 years old.

In the spring of 1990, there was a calcification change in her mammogram. In July of that year, she had a biopsy and learned it was malignant.

In August, she entered the hospital and had a lumpectomy. The pathology report showed the margins were not clear, so in September, she once again entered the hospital, this time for a simple mastectomy.

Lynne was the oldest child in a very close–knit family. She had two sisters and one brother. She had a very pleasant childhood. However, the two years prior to her diagnosis of breast cancer were very stressful. There were many changes in her life.

In the fall of 1987, her husband was transferred out of state. Lynne resigned a professional job in order to help repair her home to put it on the market—the home in which she had planned to live for the rest of her life.

In the spring of 1988, Lynne and her husband sold their home and moved. In May, she accepted a new job. The day that she accepted this job, her husband revealed to her he wanted to leave. He moved out of the house, and three months later, Lynne moved out. In December, they signed a separation agreement. The following year, in February, Lynne, along with seven other employees, was laid off from her job as a designer. Thus began an unsuccessful search for a job as a designer. She was able to get contract work—

but was without insurance coverage. Then, just about the time her divorce was finalized, she learned she had breast cancer.

At first, Lynne could not believe her diagnosis. Her first visit to the surgeon's office, however, offered her much hope, as she was told it was an "early, small, likely slow-growing type of cancer." She thought, "OK, I have a lot to do and don't want to miss any of it, so I can make it through this." Almost immediately, though, her emotions began to swing from positive thoughts to fear, shock, panic, anger, tension, and sadness. She began losing her self-confidence, having self-doubt, going through crying spells, and was unable to sleep. Her whole life seemed hopeless. As if the physical and emotional stress were not enough, she was losing control of many things due to financial loss.

Lynne felt humiliated at having to accept help from family and friends. Her illness had increased her debt and took valuable time from her career. She got behind on her obligations. This only complicated her problems. Lynne had always been such a perfectionist and did everything just right.

Cancer has changed Lynne in many ways. Physically, she is more aware of pain, due to arthritic problems. Also, she deals with a daily reminder in bathing and dressing that she has had breast cancer. However, Lynne began attending a therapy support group, where she has met many caring people. She has learned, through relaxation and visual imagery techniques, methods for improving her life. She is a more forgiving woman and more tolerant. She is once again finding new meaning in life. She looks forward to that special time each day when she can relax and be good to herself.

As a survivor, Lynne feels happy with her victory over cancer. However, it seems the insurance industry doesn't see it that way. Her insurance problem is constantly there to remind her. By the time she writes or checks "pre-existing condition," the verdict comes back "coverage denied." It seems that either insurance premiums for pre-existing conditions are so expensive she can't afford coverage or there may be a rider, meaning the company will cover everything except cancer. So, for Lynne, health insurance has been a very difficult aspect of facing cancer. However, Lynne is once again employed by a reliable company where she hopes eventually to once again have good health coverage.

For now, Lynne is alive and happy. She feels good about herself. She has regained her self–confidence and is well on her journey to recovery.

Norma: Belonging To A Therapy Support Group

I can't say enough good things about a support group for cancer survivors. After my mastectomy, radiation, and chemotherapy were finished, there did come a time when I hit that "brick wall" of feeling like I wasn't getting any help and was facing cancer totally alone.

All of my doctors were smart, skilled, and compassionate. Each one, in his or her own way, had attributes that have saved my life. I'll always be grateful to them. My family and friends were supportive, stubborn, and tireless in their efforts to care for me, especially my husband and children. Thank goodness my husband wasn't just a "fair weather sailor." You would think that with so much help from so many people, I couldn't need anything more—but I did. There were just some things I couldn't talk to them about. When I talked about my cancer, pain, or suffering, everyone withdrew. I now know they became upset and insecure when I talked about those sensitive subjects.

That's when I realized they couldn't really help me any more with this area of my recovery, and I started going to a therapy support group. Here were people who had "walked a mile in my shoes." Here were others going through the stages of denial, anger, fear, and frustration that I was experiencing. Here were people who listened with understanding and empathy. I could talk about my feelings without causing them stress or fear that I might die.

I think cancer survivors are some of the bravest people in the world. They are forced to face their own mortality in a split-second of time and then go on living. That time of great bravery came for me when, after the biopsy, the surgeon said, "I'm sorry, but it is cancer." If fear could have killed me, that is when I would have dropped dead. Like all other cancer survivors, I was forced to face death head on and do battle for my life.

Cancer forced me into going through the stages of panic, fear, disbelief, anger, and finally, acceptance— just like others had before me. Quickly, I had to find that fighting spark within my weak and sick body. I had to come to grips with the reality of the sickness, uncertainty, pain, and treatments of the disease in order to heal.

My heart became so filled with sensitivity that I cried more easily than ever before in my life. I still do, but that's OK. Tears are healing. I learned in a therapy support group that tears of sadness and happiness are both healing in their own way.

Looking back and reflecting on how bad things were in 1989 during the treatments makes me so appreciate the good times now. The changes that have taken place in my life and the adjustments I've made make me want to do more happy, useful things and to make my time count for something. I like to give words of kindness and encouragement to others now, in appreciation for all that were given to me when I needed them the most. Hearing positive words enforces the feeling that I will survive and live a rich and long life. I've learned lots of ways (thanks to support groups) to chase away the blues, depression, and fear, and to replace those feelings with joy and peace.

Don't be afraid to reach out your hand and say,

"I've been very sick. I've been hurt, physically and emotionally, help me." You'll get so much help, you won't know what to do with all of it. You'll be surprised at where, when, and from whom that help comes. It comes in so many unexpected ways, shapes, colors, and kinds that one day you'll be healed and ready to help those who reach out to you for understanding and support.

We would all like to live by the golden rule, "Do unto others as you would have them do unto you." There comes a time in everybody's life when they realize they must and can let someone help them. That's what a support group is basically all about.

I now understand the golden rule—and myself—a whole lot better. And it's just the beginning. I'll be continuing to gain knowledge, to change for the better, and to build a stronger *me* with the support of caring people. I have the support and love of my family and friends, and they certainly have my gratitude, love and support always. Plus—and this is a mighty big plus—I am a member of some wonderful support groups!

Since joining the Life After Cancer-Pathways therapy support group, I have had an attitude adjustment that has enriched my life. There, I learned that the mind can influence your health and that you can have some degree of mental control over your disease. Positive thinking can conquer pain, depression, anxiety, and lengthen your life.

The support group leaders have taught me how to

kindness and not to dwell so much on the quantity of life. The group is a warm and safe place to belong, to share the good and the bad, and to bond with others through a common problem we're trying to work out. Everyone in a support group understands what you are feeling much more than your well-meaning (but anxious) family and friends do. It is simply that everyone in the support group is fighting for his or her life, the same as you.

I'll always be grateful for the better I made in my life as a direct result of being part of a support group. I've changed so much emotionally, physically, and mentally that I no longer hide my body or my true feelings. Being part of several support groups (Life After Cancer-Pathways, Four Seasons Breast Cancer Support Group, and Reach To Recovery), has allowed me to grow, expand my horizons, and now, the sky isn't even the limit. There is no limit. I can reach higher and higher.

It is possible that, some day, I might hear those words again, "I'm sorry, but it is cancer," and I won't be afraid or alone. I'll know what to do.

I'm here today. I'm alive. I feel great and I'm not afraid of the future. I embrace it with open arms.

Polly's Story

Polly was diagnosed with ductal breast cancer in 1991, at the age of 43. Having a family history of breast cancer (her mother is a 25 year survivor), she first became concerned when her lymph nodes felt

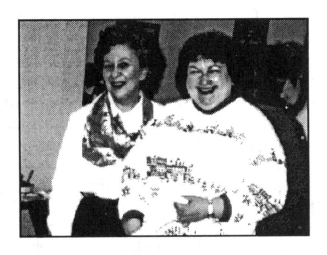

The authors at a Life After Cancer-Pathways Christmas party in 1991.

enlarged. Following a mammogram which showed no problems, her surgeon was still concerned enough to go that extra mile.

Upon learning that she had breast cancer, Polly describes her reaction then as "shock and fear." She also says, "I had a 'rock' in the pit of my stomach for about a month after surgery."

Polly's breast cancer was treated with surgery and then chemotherapy. She takes the hormonal therapy drug tamoxifen, and has so far chosen not to have reconstruction. Before the discovery of her breast cancer, she had moved to California with her family, found it wasn't right for them, and moved back to North Carolina. In her words, "That was a very stressful time for me." As is sometimes the case, stress or unusual circumstances are often experienced prior to a diagnosis of a serious illness.

Being raised in a family that believed in lots of family activities, Polly now keeps her own family and herself involved in activities that benefit them and their community. She enjoys exercising with an aerobics class, does volunteer counseling with battered women, belongs to an enrichment class, plays the guitar and sings, and is a member of a therapy support group. Of the support group she says, "I am part of Life after Cancer-Pathways, which I love. I use visualization and the relaxation techniques a good deal—great stuff."

Polly is an excellent example of a breast cancer survivor who is picking up the pieces of her life and making it even better than it was before. She is now on the road to health and happiness, both physically and mentally. During her own personal journey through the cancer experience, she has learned many wonderful truths. She shares her story to say, "Life just keeps getting better and better."

A Letter of Thanks to the Leaders at Life After Cancer–Pathways

We come to Life After Cancer-Pathways because we're fighting cancer, but that's not the only reason we stay.

We're not just fair weather sailors. By the time you meet us we've been sailing on some pretty stormy seas, physically and emotionally. Most of us feel we've been kicked around a lot and are tired, frustrated, and hurt. LAC-P is the safest port in a storm some of us have had in a long time.

We do indeed feel safe here. We know that no one is going to hurt us here. You have our trust simply because you tell us the truth. You have our respect because you treat us like we are worthwhile. You have our loyalty because you are all so committed. You have our admiration because you're all so knowledgeable. You have our love because you give love and care.

And you are all so kind! Some of the people who pass through these doors have never known such genuine kindness. Some must even learn how to respond to it.

We are getting better, both physically and emotionally, with your help and guidance. We thank you with all our hearts for all you give to us. We know you helped those here before us, and we know you will be helping all those who come here after us.

You give the most precious of gifts to us— yourselves.

--Allie Fair and Norma Suzette

Letting Go

To let go doesn't mean to stop caring—it means I can't do it for someone else.

To let go is not to cut myself off—it's the realization that I can't control another.

To let go is not to enable—but to allow learning from natural consequences.

To let go is to admit powerlessness—which means the outcome is not in my hands.

To let go is not to try to change or blame another—I can only change myself.

To let go is not to care for—but to care about.

To let go is not to fix—but to be supportive.

To let go is not to judge—but to allow another to be a human being.

To let go is not to be in the middle arranging all outcomes—but to allow others to effect their own outcomes.

To let go is not to be protective—it is to permit another to face reality.

To let go is not to deny—but to accept.

To let go is not to nag, scold, or argue—but to search out and correct my own shortcomings.

To let go is not to adjust everything to my desires—but to take each day as it comes and to cherish the moment.

To let go is not to criticize or regulate anyone—but to try to become what I dream I can be.

To let go is not to regret the past—but to grow and live for the future.

To let go is to fear less and to love more.

--Life After Cancer–Pathways Newsletter

4  THE IMMUNE SYSTEM

You've finished your treatment—surgery, chemo, radiation, whatever—and your doctor has dismissed you until your next routine check-up. You expected to be elated. Instead, you're probably bewildered, and feel as though you've lost your security blanket. Welcome to the club! But don't give up hope. There are a number of things you can do to improve your physical condition, as well as your mental state.

You can influence your immune system. Studies have shown that the average person gets cancer six times a year. According to that, we should all have cancer. Why don't we? Because our immune system is designed to fight cancer. Cancer cells are recognized by the immune system as *foreign*, and if it is working properly, it will reject them.

The thymus gland, which is located directly behind the breast bone, manufactures a number of different hormones. These hormones travel throughout the body looking for cancer cells. When they find one, they attach themselves to it and send a signal to the thymus gland. The thymus gland then sends out thousands of natural killer cells (known as *T-cells*), which go directly to the cancer cell and kill it, then return to the thymus gland until needed again.

Until the 1970s, doctors usually believed that the brain and the immune system worked independently of each other. Then it was discovered that nerve fibers in the thymus gland produced these "immune cells" known as T-cells. Because all nerves are connected in some way to the brain, researchers began to pay more attention to the link between the brain and the immune system.

The secret is to keep the immune system in good working order. Many things influence the immune system. Stress, depression, anxiety, and emotional problems can lower its ability to function properly. Studies have shown that a large number of women who have breast cancer developed it within two years after the death of their husbands.

There are many ways to improve the effectiveness of the immune system, most of them involving common sense and a good life style. Good nutrition is important, also rest and sleep, exercise, humor, coping with stress, and, above all, a positive attitude. A recent study showed that people who had pets or plants to care for recuperated from illness faster than those who did not.

Good Nutrition

Good nutrition is important to everyone, but particularly to the cancer survivor. Learn all you can about the basic food groups and use your willpower to eat a well-balanced diet.

Skip the fast food route. Instead, take time to eat a real meal. Preserved or pickled foods may contain nitrates, which can be changed into carcinogens. Other foods favor the growth of cancer. These include fat and alcohol.

By making wise eating choices, you may be able to fortify your natural defenses and prevent many of the problems caused by an immune system breakdown. Some foods, such as fruits, vegetables, and whole grains, actually help prevent cancer. The best plan is to eat a variety of foods, maintain a healthy weight, eat a low–fat diet (avoid saturated fats and cholesterol), eat plenty of fruit, vegetables, and grains, and use sugar, salt, sodium, and alcohol in moderation.

The following nutrients are thought to build the immune system:

Beta carotene: Protects against cancer; maintains healthy skin and mucous membranes--which protect against invasion by infectious organisms. Found in carrots, sweet potatoes, spinach, cantaloupes, apricots, broccoli, peaches, cherries, tomatoes, and liver.

Vitamin C: Can improve immunity against viruses, and may help fight cancer. Found in green peppers, broccoli, Brussels sprouts, cauliflower, strawberries, citrus fruits, cantaloupes, papaya.

Vitamin E: Stimulates the immune system. Found in dark green vegetables, eggs, liver, wheat germ, vegetable oils, and peanuts.

Iron: Promotes resistance to stress and disease. Found in liver, prunes, eggs, peas, oysters, raisins, and artichokes.

Selenium: Protects against carcinogens. Found in butter, bran, celery, whole apple cider, vinegar, fish, and legumes.

(Above is based on information from the book Maximum Immunity *by Michael A. Weiner.)*

Relaxation

Stress is probably the worst enemy of the immune system. Studies have proved that stress lowers our ability to fight disease—and *that* is when the cancer cells in the body have a chance to get a head start. Relaxation builds the immune system and enables the T-cells to be more active. There are numerous ways to practice relaxation. It is often taught and practiced in therapy support groups, but can easily be done at home alone. It is a technique that has to be learned, and it's possible to become quite adept at it in a short time.

Try this process: First, get in a comfortable position in a quiet place, where you will not be interrupted. Close your eyes and focus on your breathing. As you take deep, slow breaths, think of the incoming breath bringing in relaxation and the out breath releasing tension, stress, and any problems or worries you may have.

Visualize yourself in one of your favorite places—

Visualize yourself in one of your favorite places—at the beach, in a beautiful mountain setting, a garden, any place you have been, or even a place you just made up. Be aware of the scenery, the colors, the textures, smells and sounds. Just enjoy being there, thinking happy thoughts.

When they are thoroughly relaxed, some people envision their T-cells going all through the body, seeking out cancer cells and attacking them. They may picture the T–cells as guard dogs, a battalion of Marines, Pac-men, piranhas, or any creative thing that has meaning for you.

There are many cassette tapes available to help you with the relaxation process. Carl Simonton did a tape called *Relaxation and Mental Imagery.* There are also some excellent ones by Lawrence LeShan, Bernie Siegel, Louise Hay, Joan Boryshenko, and many others. You might also want to try tapes of relaxing music and nature sounds. Whatever works best for you is fine.

Take time out for this relaxation exercise several times a week. You'll be amazed at the difference it will make in your life. You'll be more relaxed physically and mentally, plus have more energy and ability to cope with the stresses of life. Sounds like a formula that's hard to beat—so why wait?

Rest and Sleep

The idea of relaxation leads naturally into the subject of rest and sleep. Before you had cancer, you may never have thought of resting during the day, and sleep at night was something you did only when everything you needed or wanted to do was finished. If that was the case, you really need to revise your life style. If you use all your energy this way, your body won't have anything left for the immune system. The major organs—such as the brain, the lungs, and the heart—get their share first. The immune system is last, and consequently, it gets fed best while the other organs are at rest.

Taking out a few minutes for relaxation, several times during the day, will do wonders. Use your relaxation techniques; literally take time to smell the roses. Sit and meditate for a few minutes, or listen to your favorite music. And always, always get a good night's sleep.

Exercise

Exercise is vital to your physical well-being. Fortunately, in the world today there is more emphasis on physical fitness than there was a few decades ago. Many people are into jogging, aerobics, and walking. Your choice is limited only by your physical capacity. If it makes you feel exhilarated, it's good for you; if you're completely exhausted, you've overdone it.

If you happen to be a couch potato, or are limited by your working hours, there is a relatively painless way to exercise. Walk as vigorously as possible when going from the office to the bank or post office, and take a few minutes during your lunch hour to walk around a few blocks. When going to the grocery store or mall, don't try to find the closest parking place. Instead, park as far away from the entrance as possible and get in a little exercise in walking. You can also put in a little extra mileage while doing your shopping. If you're away from home, take a walking tour around an interesting city.

Humor

Humor does wonders for the immune system, as well as making life more enjoyable. The value of humor is not new. In Proverbs 15:13 we find, "A merry heart maketh a cheerful countenance, but by sorrow the spirit is broken." A good laugh does wonders for morale. Learn to look for the humor in every situation—everything is not always gloom and doom.

Try a few of the following suggestions for how to create more humor in your everyday life. Read funny books and watch funny movies. Everyone has their favorites that they identify with. Clip cartoons and jokes you enjoy from newspapers and magazines and then share them with others. Be more playful. Play with your children, grandchildren, and pets more. Practice new jokes you hear, if you like them, and tell them to other people.

Positive Attitude

Another of your greatest assets is a positive atti-tude. It can influence your recovery time and enhance the quality of your life. A positive, upbeat attitude does not always happen automatically. Sometimes you have it, and other times you have to work at it. Refuse to think negative thoughts about yourself and others. Educate yourself by reading self-help books and listening to self-help and inspirational cassette tapes. Be around only people who have positive attitudes. Learn to express the best that is in you and choose to be happy and healthy.

Try using affirmations. Affirmations are positive thoughts that you consciously focus on in order to obtain a desired result. They can be used whenever you wish to bring some good into your life.

Remember—a truly happy, well rested, well nourished, and responsible person has a strong immune system. It really is your choice.

Home Instruction: Post- Mastectomy Exercises

These are some of the exercises we found especially helpful during our recovery process. You should immediately begin to use the arm affected by your surgery in personal hygiene (such as washing your face, combing your hair, brushing your teeth, and dressing). These, exercises, designed to strengthen, repair, and rehabilitate problem shoulders, are some of many exercises available. These are reprinted with permission from Professional Care Systems. Always check with your doctor or physical therapist before beginning any exercise program.

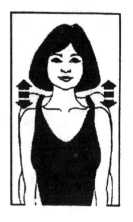

Shoulder Shrug

Shrug the shoulders upward and downward for flexibility. Pull the shoulders backward while pushing chest upward.

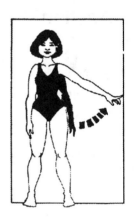

Walk Up the Wall—for flexibility

a. Stand adjacent to the wall, so that fingertips touch the wall.

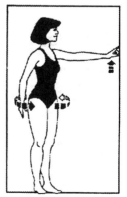

b. As fingers move upward, gradually turn torso to the wall.

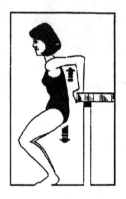

Deep Knee Bend

Lower body slowly to a deep knee bend, using a table for support.

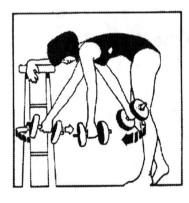

Shoulder Traction Exercise

Rest head comfortably on stool or counter. Holding a two to five pound weight, book, or can of food, allow arm to swing freely.

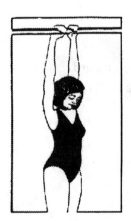

Spinal Traction Exercise

Hang from bar suspended in a doorway.

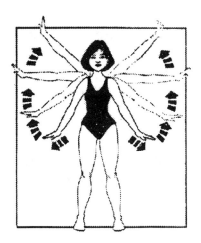

Trunk and Shoulder Stretch

Push outward while lifting arms over head. Repeat with downward movement.

Take Care Of Yourself!

The most important thing to remember is no one is going to take care of you like you! Be your own best friend. Here are some ways I do this:

Flowers for me: Most of us enjoy flowers. It's so exciting to receive a bouquet—pink, yellow, or red roses, yellow daisies, or purple violets—but you don't have to wait for someone to send you flowers; get some for yourself! A friend recently told me that quite frequently, she had a single rose delivered to her-self—and enjoyed it tremendously. This is being good to yourself. You deserve a rose today. Enjoy!

My personal journal: Keeping a journal of my feelings and thoughts helped me. There were days when I did not want to write anything. Other days, I would write page after page in my journal. Months later, as I read from my journal, I was finally able to deal with those things. I didn't hurt when I read and thought about those problems. Sometimes, I could even smile about the topics. I would highly recommend that a person get a blank book and write for fifteen minutes a day. Just write what you are feeling and why. This will be your journal—yours to keep, to read, to cry over, and maybe even smile over. Researchers say that keeping a journal enhances the immune system.

POST-MASTECTOMY LYMPHEDEMA

What is *lymphedema*? How, where, when, and why does it affect breast cancer survivors? What can you do to avoid getting it—and if you do get lymphedema, how do you treat it? Here are the facts about this disease, followed by personal stories of women who have it.

Most breast cancer patients, if they have had surgery, radiation therapy, node dissections, or a combination of these treatments, are at high risk for lymphedema. There are many causes for this disease, different stages, and several types of treatment. We are concentrating only on the type of lymphedema that might affect breast cancer patients. This is called *secondary lymphedema,* and can be *acute* or *chronic. Acute lymphedema* is a temporary condition following radical surgery with nodal dissections and/or radiation and only lasts for a short time (a few days). *Chronic lymphedema* is a long term condition.

Lymphedema is defined as *the accumulation of*

excess lymph fluid and proteins in the interstitial spaces, principally of the subcutaneous fat, caused by a fault in the lymphatic system. Secondary lymphedema, the lymphedema experienced by oncology patients, *is due to involvement of the lymph nodes or vessels by cancer, or to surgical or radiation effects on the lymphatics draining dependent areas of the body.* In short, your arm swells.

Chronic lymphedema is a progressive, and usually permanent, disease. Initial swelling may be slow and gradual, or may progress very rapidly. Its natural progression leads to a progressive increase in the size of the affected limb, which may lead to occupational disability, social disability due to clothing restrictions, increasing frequency of infections (*cellulitis*) of the affected limb, and increasing difficulty in managing episodes of skin breakdown problems. Although somewhat rare, the disease may ultimately lead to amputation when infection becomes resistant to drug therapy.

Post-mastectomy lymphedema usually occurs from one to five years after the operation, but it can actually occur at any time after breast cancer treatments. This chronic swelling of the arm may affect only the arm above the elbow or the whole arm and hand. Chronic lymphedema in breast cancer survivors is a significant long term complication resulting in physical discomfort, debilitation, and cosmetic disfigurement.

When lymphedema begins, one usually notices

swelling of the arm or hand. A ring may seem tighter on the finger or a favorite blouse may seem too tight around the arm. Sometimes pain or a feeling of "pins and needles" may result. When you notice any of these symptoms, it is very important to seek medical advice. If the problem is diagnosed and treatment begins early, the chances of reversing the condition is much greater than if the swelling is ignored.

When lymphedema remains untreated, or when it progresses rapidly, the lymph vessels and tissue become harder and less elastic, resulting in *"hard" lymphedema*. "Hard" lymphedema may be the result of collagen build up or of scar tissue from repeated swelling or repeated infections, and is the most difficult to reverse.

What Is the Lymphatic System?

Lymph is a transparent, usually slightly yellow, often opalescent liquid found within the lymphatic vessels. This liquid is collected from tissues in all parts of the body and returned to the blood via the lymphatic system. If your lymphatic system has been damaged (radiation) or removed (mastectomy), then the deficient lymphatic system of the arm is incapable of compensating for the increased demand for drainage of fluid. Sometimes, cancer itself can spread to the lymph nodes, causing an interruption of the normal lymphatic pathway and pooling of fluid.

The lymphatic system in our bodies is a very

important part of the normal circulatory system, which also includes veins and arteries. The purpose of the lymphatic system is to produce cells of the immune system that help fight bacteria and viruses. The lymph vessels (or channels) contain the lymph fluid. The lymph nodes are "stations" of the lymph system. All lymph fluid passing through these stations (or valves) is purified of waste matter, and bacteria and viruses are made harmless. That's a tall order!

Early in the course of developing lymphedema, the patient will experience soft, pitting edema (swelling) that is easily improved by elevation and elastic support. Continual and progressive lymphedema, however, causes dilation of the lymph vessels and backflow of fluid to the tissue beds where lymph pores are pulled open. This allows lymph fluid (which is rich in protein) to remain in the tissue of the arm longer, creating a favorable environment for the growth of bacteria and the possibility of infection. The tissue also has a lower oxygen content, which allows stagnant fluid to interfere with healing.

Since there is no other route for tissue protein (albumin) transport to the vascular space, there are very few effective treatments for advanced lymphedema. Additionally, once these tissues are stretched, edema recurs much more readily. This is why it is so important that breast cancer survivors get adequate information about lymphedema!

The Normal Lymphatic System

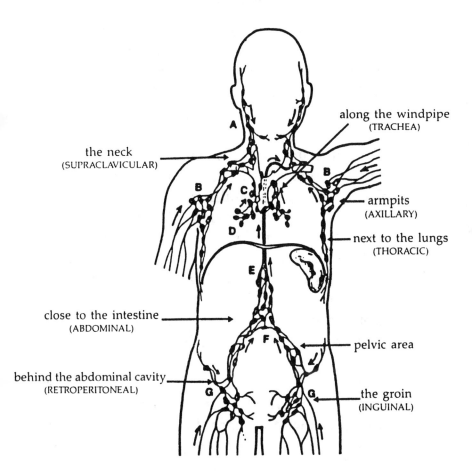

along the windpipe
(TRACHEA)

the neck
(SUPRACLAVICULAR)

armpits
(AXILLARY)

next to the lungs
(THORACIC)

close to the intestine
(ABDOMINAL)

pelvic area

behind the abdominal cavity
(RETROPERITONEAL)

the groin
(INGUINAL)

(Illustration from *Lymphedema: General Information.*" Reprinted by permission of C.B.F., Inc. Call 1-800-225-8129 for additional information about Lymphedema.)

Do's and Dont's for Prevention and Control of Lymphedema

1. Elevate the affected arm (above the level of the heart) whenever possible to improve the circulation of the weakened system.
2. Avoid heavy lifting with the affected arm, as this puts strain on the arm with poor circulation.
3. Avoid vigorous, repetitive movements or resistance against the affected arm (rubbing, scrubbing, pushing, or pulling objects). Physical exertion causes the blood to flow more rapidly through the muscle and tissue. Some blood will be absorbed by the tissue and the lymphatic system, making the lymphatic system work harder than it is capable of doing.
4. Avoid rapid, circular movements that cause gravity to pull fluid centrifugally toward the hand.
5. Check with your physician about any sports activities in which you participate. Again, physical exertion causes the lymphatic system to work harder than it is capable of, aggravating the condition.
6. Wear gloves while doing housework, gardening, or other types of work that can result in even minor injuries. Any injury that would open the skin could provide an opportunity for infection.
7. Wear thimbles when sewing.

8. *Never* allow injection or blood drawing in the affected arm! Again, piercing the skin provides an entry for infection.

9. Use an electric razor rather than a razor blade.

10. Avoid cutting cuticles when manicuring the hands.

11. *Avoid* insect bites! If bitten by an insect (or scratched by a pet) on the affected arm, seek medical attention at once. This is very important to prevent a serious infection.

12. Use hypoallergenic soap, deodorant, and lubricants. Good hygiene keeps the skin clean and dry and protected from irritation and potential infection. Avoid harsh chemicals.

13. Clean breaks in the skin with soap and water, then use an antibacterial ointment. (Use gauze wrapping instead of tape.)

14. Consult your doctor if you develop a rash (or blisters).

15. Keep the affected arm protected from the sun. Sunbathing is risky, since heat tends to increase blood flow through the tissue, thereby overworking the lymphatic system.

16. Avoid extreme temperature changes (hot and cold) when bathing, washing dishes, cooking, etc. Sensation in the affected arm may be diminished.

17. Avoid constrictive pressure on the affected arm and hand. Wearing tight clothing and jewelry would worsen the circulation that is

already impaired.

18. Do not have blood pressure checked on the affected arm. The inflated blood pressure cuff further limits the circulation in an arm that already has poor circulation.

19. Carry your handbag on the unaffected arm or shoulder.

20. If your prosthesis is large, make sure it is lightweight. Heavy breast prostheses used after mastectomy may put too much pressure on lymph nodes above the collar bone, thereby slowing and interrupting the pathway of the lymphatic system.

21. Be sure to eat a well-balanced, low–salt, protein-rich diet. This will help you to avoid excess weight or fluid in the arm.

22. Watch for signs of infection (redness, pain, heat, swelling, fever) and report them to your doctor immediately! Other signs to watch for (and report) are feelings of tightness, decreased strength, aching, heaviness, and numbness.

23. Also, immediately report to your doctor any sudden increase in the size of your arm or hand. Early management of the swelling may stem or delay fibrosis, severe debilitation, and immobility.

Baby that arm! Watch it closely for any changes, treat it gently, don't abuse it by overworking it, protect it from harm, and most of all—just love and appreciate it for all of the things it does for you every day!

NOTE: Post-mastectomy exercises prescribed by your physician or physical therapist are generally not considered harmful to your arm and hand. Isometric exercises may be helpful.

Treatments for Lymphedema

The treatment plan for lymphedema will, of course, depend on the actual cause, the type, and the stage of the disease. It is important to remember that lymphedema can occur at any time (even as late as fifteen years) after treatments for breast cancer. Breast cancer survivors who are well informed and practice good hygiene, good nutrition, and appropriate exercise show a significantly lower incidence of lymphedema.

Contributing factors for each individual case of lymphedema should be assessed, evaluated, and monitored. These factors may include the following: nutritional status, obesity, immobility, and a history of other medical conditions, such as edema, prior radiation or surgery, diabetes, hypertension, kidney disease, cardiac disease, or phlebitis. Every breast cancer survivor should understand the hazards of lymphedema and know that lifelong vigilance is needed to care for the affected arm.

Acute Lymphedema

Acute lymphedema (post-mastectomy) is a temporary condition that may occur for approximately four to six days following radical surgical procedures with associated nodal dissections. The following factors place the patient at risk for acute lymphedema: surgical drains, inflammation, immobility, infection, removal of lymph nodes, and radiation. Acute lymphedema must be monitored and regulated very closely in the immediate postoperative period to avoid further complications.

Acute lymphedema is treated by keeping the arm elevated as much as possible, pressure (using an elastic compression sleeve), exercise (as prescribed), and manual lymph drainage treatments. The manual lymph drainage treatments are done by a physical therapist specially trained in the type of massage that pushes the lymph fluid out of the arm and also stimulates the remaining lymph vessels.

It is also important with acute lymphedema that other factors be taken into account, because massage and techniques to encourage drainage would be harmful if there was a blockage in the arm. There are special tests (such as lymph node scans and venograms) to determine if any lymph or blood vessel blockage exists.

Exercise is helpful in the prevention and cure of acute lymphedema. Breast cancer patients should be instructed about proper hand and arm exercises after mastectomy. How soon the exercise is started following surgery and/or radiation should be the decision of your physician or physical therapist.

The recovery rate for acute lymphedema is increased when it is detected and treated early.

1. Elevation. Elevating the arm above the heart (wrist joint above the elbow, elbow joint above the shoulder joint) improves the circulation and drainage with the help of gravity.

2. Pressure. The proper amount of pressure applied to the arm and hand by elastic compression sleeves (bandages) reduces and controls the swelling.

3. Exercise. Lymphatic drainage is improved when exercising muscles squeeze the soft tissue and force excess fluid into the blood stream. Check with your doctor or physical therapist for safe, effective exercises.

4. Massage. Manual treatment pushes the extra lymph fluid out of the arm and stimulates the remaining lymph vessels.

5. Remember the "Do's and Dont's."

NOTE: Diuretics (fluid pills) should be used with caution. Most diuretics encourage vascular fluid depletion, but do nothing for excess protein deposits and could hasten connective tissue fibrosis. Also, tamoxifen may cause some edema (swelling).

Infection

If lymphedema is caused by an infection, your

doctor will prescribe the appropriate antibiotics.

Infection may be a serious problem at any time following surgery, radiation, and chemotherapy. It is important to diagnose the specific type of infection (that is, fungal, gram positive cocci) with a blood test (CBC) and begin treatment immediately. Infection in the arm or body may cause edema, and may lead to an increase of protein deposits in the tissues, cellulitis, or fibrosis of the affected arm. *Cellulitis* is inflammation of cellular tissue, especially loose connective tissue next to the skin. *Fibrosis* is an increase in the fibrinogen and fibroblasts in the connective tissue (scarring and hardening).

Remember the signs of infection—such as, redness, pain, heat, swelling, fever, and blisters. Report any of these signs to a doctor.

Always carry antibiotics or a prescription for antibiotics with you. Repeated infections may cause scarring and hardening of the tissues in the arm. This makes the progression toward chronic lymphedema more likely. Review the section on "Do's and Dont's."

Chronic Lymphedema

Chronic lymphedema is the most difficult of all types of edema to reverse. Due to its nature, a vicious and persistent cycle is started, wherein the deficient lymphatic system of the arm is unable to handle the overload of fluid.

Chronic lymphedema, after a time, no longer

responds to elevation, elastic compression devices, or any of the other methods for treating temporary lymphedema. The swollen tissues of the arm are less well–nourished and more prone to necrosis (death) during immobility. Therefore, it is important to watch for areas of skin breakdown, especially over bony prominences, such as your knuckles and elbow.

The vicious and constant cycle of swelling, infections, and injury—swelling, infections, and injury, repeatedly stretch, scar, and harden every cell in the affected arm. The lymphatic system (being damaged) can no longer do its job of protecting and cleansing the arm in the face of this overwhelming cycle. Accumulation of collagen proteins, inflammation, fibrosis of the connective tissue, and retention of excessive amounts of fluid all cause the arm to become larger.

As the arm grows in size, the brawny, stiff, non-pitting appearance of chronic lymphedema becomes evident. The arm (and sometimes the hand) may become twice the normal size (or even larger) and may be permanently disfigured. This may (understandably) cause depression in some women, as they develop an altered body image.

With chronic lymphedema, the arm naturally becomes heavier and may cause problems in the shoulder, neck, and back. The body has to adjust to carrying and balancing the extra weight. Some women experience pain as a result of pressure on the nerve endings, making normal, everyday movements more difficult. This heaviness, pain, and disfigurement is stressful enough on its own, without it being there as a constant reminder to you that you have survived breast cancer and its treatments!

Women with chronic lymphedema are less likely to improve their functional status and mobility without help. Proper treatment and therapy is essential to learning to live with the disability of this disease.

Prior to beginning treatments for chronic lymphedema, the following information may be helpful in assessing, preventing, and treating some symptoms:

Physical Pain may be managed using non-narcotic analgesics, relaxation techniques, mild to strong narcotic analgesics, adjuvant drugs (like Elavil) and/or superficial stimulation.

Emotional Pain may be helped by health care professionals, encouragement from family and friends, or a support group where a woman can vent her concerns and fears.

Thrombosis (blood clots) may be managed with anticoagulation therapy. These clots could cause serious circulatory and respiratory problems if they are not eliminated by medication prior to treatments.

Disability may require assistance with the activities of daily living at home and on the job. The functional level (which includes strength, agility, and sensitivity) of the arm is impaired.

Deterioration of the arm may be prevented and/ or slowed by following the treatment plan that is correct for your stage of chronic lymphedema. It would be negligent to minimize the symptoms or to underestimate the progression of the disease.

Current Treatments for Chronic Lymphedema

Before presenting the methods of treatment currently available for chronic lymphedema, it must be stressed that all of the preceding information regarding acute lymphedema, infections, and especially the "Do's and Dont's for Prevention and Control," also apply to the woman suffering from chronic lymphedema.

Also, remember that only your physician, who has a complete medical history about you, can help you determine what care and methods of treatment are advisable in your case.

Learning to live with chronic lymphedema takes first, the proper medical treatment, and second, patience, common sense, diligence, and adequate information. A meticulous skin care regime is also important. So have hope—there is help!

1. Sequential Gradient Pump

The sequential gradient pump is a devise that works using physiological (characteristic of normal or natural) principles. Pressure is distributed into air compartments which are contained in a special sleeve. The sleeve fits over (envelops) the affected arm and the compartments are sequentially (following in order) inflated. The pump cycle starts by filling the distal compartment first (hand) and continues inflating the remaining compartments in sequence toward the proximal compartment (shoulder), thereby pressing the fluid up and out of the arm. The overlapping compartments prevent any gaps between the functioning compartments to achieve a maximal reduction of the edema (swelling).

Actual frequency, duration, and pressure of therapy using the pump may be determined by your physician or health care professional.

There are some women who *cannot* use the pump. Contraindications for use include deep venous thrombosis, acute infections of the affected arm, decompensated cardiac failure (arterial insufficiency), or other problems diagnosed by a physician.

Women who do use the pump find it to be very helpful in reducing the amount of fluid in the arm, thus reducing the size of the arm. It also relieves pain (caused by the swelling) and helps improve circulation. Reduction in arm size and relief of pain are very important to someone with chronic lymphedema!

Treatment with the sequential pneumatic pump can even be done at home after the patient has been trained to operate the pump.

2. Elastic Compression Sleeves

Elastic compression sleeves are worn on the arm

(and hand) to apply pressure and thus reduce and/or control the swelling. Appropriate strength compression sleeves may be prescribed by your physician and fitted by a health care professional. Gloves that provide pressure for the hand and fingers are available, and may be custom-fitted. Sleeves do come in fashion colors.

Elastic compression sleeves are used in conjunction with the pneumatic pump, and are usually worn after a pump down and during ambulation (normal activity). The following tips will help you develop a good "relationship" with your elastic sleeve:

1. Wear only clean sleeves over clean skin. Soiled garments not only compromise the skin, but skin oils and dirt buildup will break down the resilience of the fiber. Sleeves must be hand washed with very mild liquid soap, rinsed well, and air dried.

2. Have two sleeves so that you can alternate them on a daily basis. This will prolong the life of the garments, which last approximately six months.

3. Apply the sleeve in the morning before the arm has a chance to swell. Do not wear the sleeve when you retire at night.

4. A well-fitting, properly measured sleeve should be smooth, as wrinkles can cause irritation.

5. If a mild irritation develops in the elbow, a silk lining can be custom-made, or a thin foam pad can be placed there.

6. If you are under treatment, you will need to be remeasured and refitted for progressively smaller sleeves as your swelling lessens.
7. Do not wear the sleeve if there is any sign of an infection, such as a rash, redness, inflammation, pain, or fever.

3. Surgery

Surgery is not generally successful in curing lymphedema, especially in the oncology patient. If chronic lymphedema progresses to the point of being *gross* or it no longer responds to the treatments already described, it would be practical to discuss surgery with a specialist.

Surgery is seldom done in the United States at present and requires diagnostic tests beforehand. These tests, such as a lymph node scan, lymphangioscintigraphy, venogram, and MRI, determine if there is any blockage in the vessels of the affected arm.

Insurance

Most private insurance companies and Medicare provide reimbursement for procedures and therapy used to treat lymphedema, as long as they are medically necessary and prescribed by a physician.

Elastic compression garments (sleeves) and compression therapy (pneumatic pump) are usually covered by most insurance companies and Medicare, Manual lymph drainage (massage) is not usually covered. It is advisable to discuss coverage with your insurance company.

Hopefully, the general information about lymphedema that has been presented here will help you to better understanding its causes, prevention, and treatment. Just remember to love that arm (even though it may look different now) and don't be ashamed of it. Give it, and yourself, lots of TLC.

Reference List Of Garment & Pump Manufacturers*

Garments

Maker	Product	Contact
JUZO P.O. Box 1088 Cuyahoga Falls, OH 44223-0088 Telephone: (800)222-4999	Stockings & Sleeves	Gerda or Barbara
SIGVARIS P.O. Box 570 Branford, CT 06405 Telephone: (800)322-7744	Stockings & Sleeves	Bonnie
BARTON CAREY P.O. Box 421 Perryburg, OH 43551 Telephone: (800)421-0444	Custom Stockings & Sleeves	Freddie or any Sales- person
MEDI 76 West Seegers Rd. Arlington Heights, IL 60005 Telephone: (800)633-6334	Stockings & Sleeves	Customer Service
BEIERSDORF, INC. BDF Plaza Norwalk, CT 06856 Telephone: (800)648-3202 x8466	Bandages & Padding	Ruth Jossa

Pumps

Maker	Product	Contact
WRIGHT LINEAR PUMP, INC. 185A Robinson Road Imperial, PA 15126 Telephone: (800)631-9535	Pump & Custom Garments	Sandy
BIO COMPRESSION 736 Gotham Parkway Carlstadt, NJ 07072 Telephone: (800)888-0908	Sequential Circulator	Donald Warren

If your local medical supply house does not stock these garments, we suggest you call the companies listed above for the name of a local distributor.

Reprinted by permission of the National Lymphedema Network

Contacts

For more information, contact:

NATIONAL LYMPHEDEMA NETWORK
2211 Post Street, Suite 404
San Francisco, CA 94115
TEL: 800-541-3259
FAX: 415-921-4284

References

Post-mastectomy Lymphedema, The Cancer Information Service, call "1-800-4-CANCER."

Thiadens, Saskia R.J., R.N., *Lymphedema: General Information*, National Lymphedema Network Booklet, 1991. Write to the National Lymphadema Network or call 800-541-3259.

Lympha Press, *Protocol Manual*, distributed by Camp International, 1989. Write: Camp International, Inc., World Headquarters, Jackson, MI 49204-0089, or call 800-492-1088.

Benedet, Rosalind, R.N.C., M.S.N., "Compression Sleeves: The Proper Fit," *NLN Newsletter*, Volume 3, No. 2, April, 1991.

For reprints of the list on the preceding pages, request the "Reference List of Garment & Pump Manufacturers 1991" from the National Lymphedema Network.

6  LYMPHEDEMA: PERSONAL STORIES

Norma's Right Arm

My problems started immediately after radiation. My arm became red and swollen so quickly that I thought it was going to burst. The pain was a hot, heavy, aching kind of pain that stayed with me for several months. I have occasional pain now, and once or twice a year I may have an infection.

At my final appointment with the radiologist, I showed my hand to him, and after a look of despair— on his face, not mine—he said I should sleep with my arm propped up with pillows at night and perhaps learn to use my left hand more.

When I showed my swollen hand and arm to the surgeon, he said that he didn't think the surgery alone had caused the condition. I asked him what I could do to get rid of it, and that is when I began to really learn the truth about lymphedema.

I even asked the surgeon months later if he could do another surgery and reconnect the little network of lymph channels. He said *no*. Neither one of these fine doctors caused the condition. I know that now, but at the time, all I wanted was *help!*

The first help I received for the lymphedema was an elastic compression sleeve. I was given a prescription for one with the gauntlet that didn't cover the fingers, but just went across the palm and around the thumb. It didn't help at all, because it squished so much fluid down into my fingers that they turned red and were very swollen.

Other advice I was given during that first year was to keep my arm up as much as possible. This isn't always easy to do. I tried to keep it up when resting, prop it up against walls at other times, hold on to seat belts above my head, twiddle my hair, exercise, and so forth to let gravity help drain the fluid. Through all of this trial and error period, my arm kept swelling and getting bigger.

The thing that frustrated me the most was that I didn't know what to do. I wasn't getting much information on what to do or even what was available to me. By reading on my own, getting information from the American Cancer Society 1-800 number, and by reading books from the library and any other information I could get my hands on, I discovered that lymphedema is progressive, irreversible, permanent, and sometimes dangerous. Of course this alarmed me, and I began to look for better and different information.

While looking at other lymphedema sleeves at a prosthesis center, I noticed custom fitted gloves, but they told me they were for burn patients. I said, "Well, I think they'll work for my lymphedema." By being persistent, I was able to get copies of the information and pictures of the glove. These I gave to the surgeon, and he wrote me a prescription for a custom fitted elastic compression sleeve and glove. At a local drugstore, I was measured and fitted and then waited a few weeks for the items to arrive. Then I began to wear the sleeve and glove. After wearing it for a couple of hours, my arm and hand did feel better. Until I became used to wearing them all day, I sometimes felt nauseous and it did chafe my skin.

Also, I didn't know until over a year later, after my lymphedema first appeared, that if I got a bug bite, I was supposed to go to the emergency room (or that I could even get infections in that arm and needed antibiotics). I didn't know any of this, as none of this information was made available to me in the first few months of my having the condition.

I was, however, persistent—like the squeaky wheel that gets the grease—and treated myself using information I read in books and heard from other women.

After joining a support group in the spring of 1990, one of the counselors was thoughtful enough to give me the *National Lymphedema Network Newsletter*, which had a 1-800 number and an address. Eureka! I now had information galore at my fingertips. I actually corresponded with a lymphedema clinic in Atlanta, Georgia, and got more information.

I first learned about the sequential pneumatic

pumps available to people with lymphedema from the National Lymphedema Network (NLN). This valuable information has changed my life for the better. Of course I wanted my very own arm pump.

I had changed surgeons at this time, and when next I visited my new surgeon, I showed him the NLN newsletter. I was so excited about the pump, and was thrilled when he knew about them and actually showed me the one in his office. It was the first time I had ever seen one.

I ask for a prescription for an arm pump and he wrote me two prescriptions. I wanted to shop around, at his suggestion, and get the best one for me. He said, "Go for the Cadillac." The first pump I had was a slow press that had three compartments. I used it for a month and it did help the joint pain. When my arm was very swollen, it would feel hot and heavy and ache, so this pump relieved the pain—and that was wonderful to me.

The other machine that I was looking for, I finally found through another distributor. The woman there found a local representative who came and demonstrated the Lymphopress by Camp to me. It has many pressure chambers and works like a centipede walking up your arm, with pressure that "milks" your arm. In order for the insurance company to let me have the pump, I had to do a three-day "pump-down," four hours on, 30 minutes off, continuously for 72 hours, measuring every four hours. It was very painful to do it. The surgeon gave me pain pills to take while I did the pump-down.

I began to put small bandages on the ends of my fingers, where the cuticles were being pulled back, and on some of my knuckles that were beginning to look bruised or feel raw. I had lots of little broken capillaries. I even fainted once, but I was persistent. I finished the 72-hour pump-down with the measurements every four hours, even in the middle of the night. I used a high pressure during the day and a lower pressure at night while I was supposed to be sleeping—although I didn't get much sleep. But now I have the machine, which is state of the art technology, because the insurance company bought it for me. I'm so happy to have it, because it does relieve the pain and it does keep my arm smaller. Another benefit of the machine is purely psychological. I don't feel like a little, bitty woman attached to a great big arm anymore.

A woman I have talked to used an old-fashioned pump with only one compartment for almost two years. She used it three and four times a day, fifteen to twenty minutes each time. She had a routine she followed morning, noon, and night, and at other times when her arm was more swollen. She did this for almost two years. Her lymphedema totally went away and has not recurred in years.

I am now using my arm pump on a regular basis because it relieves the pain, keeps my arm and hand smaller, and also keeps my arm healthier. My arm pump means more to me than a box of diamonds.

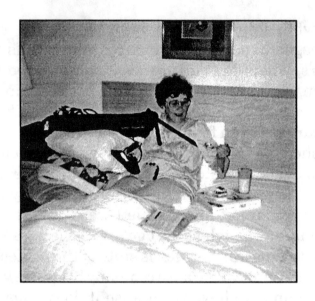

The co-author of this book, Norma Suzette Jones, with her arm pump at the beach in 1991. She says, "While using my arm pump, I can watch TV, talk on the phone, listen to tapes, read, and eat. . .all at the same time! I just haven't learned to write left–handed yet."

Miriam's Experience

It was July 21, 1969, when I opened my eyes in a Miami Hospital. Looking at the TV, I saw that the astronauts had landed on the moon—taking one giant step for mankind. My first reaction was, "Where am I and what am I doing here?" I knew I was not on the moon! I tried to remember and, of course, it all came back to me—slowly, but vividly.

I had discovered a lump in my left breast. I had

tried to brush it off—not the lump, but the idea of what it might mean. I remembered that my dog, a large one, had jumped on me and hit my chest in the exact spot as the lump. I also remembered that a tightly sprung screen door had snapped and hit the same spot. I wondered, at the time, if I should have the lump checked out or ignore it. Common sense made me choose the right course and I knew I would have it checked out.

I went to a surgeon we had used before, only to find he was out of town. His associate examined me and refused to use a needle to withdraw any fluid for determining whether or not it was cancer. He just said he wouldn't touch it. I decided to wait the two weeks for the surgeon we knew to return. Meanwhile, I called my girlfriend (who went bananas about my waiting), and she suggested that I call this doctor who was considered the best—a doctor's doctor.

Following her advice, I went to see him the next day. I remember it was a Thursday—and he put me in the hospital that same afternoon. The doctor said they would do a biopsy the next morning. Was he talking to me? Sure, there wasn't anyone else in his office, so it had to be me. Oh well, there I was in the hospital, and Friday morning they did the biopsy, afterwards telling me they were doing a 24–hour freeze section.

The doctor came in very early Saturday morning and told me it was malignant. He then told me that

I would be going in for more surgery in about two hours time. I was furious! Not because it was malignant, but because I had to go through more surgery. I remember asking him why he hadn't done it all yesterday and he responded with, "That's what they all say."

The mastectomy was performed on Saturday morning, and it was Sunday morning when I realized that the astronauts and I had both gone to the moon. My next reaction may sound trite, but in my head I said to myself, "Well, I've got two arms, two legs, and two breasts—if I had to lose one of them, I'm lucky it was a breast."

They also wanted to do an ovectomy within two days (the OB/GYN's decision), but the surgeon told them that my hormone level had dropped to almost zero and he did not think it was necessary. I had also lost a lot of blood and I guess they were afraid to do another surgery so soon after the mastectomy. You see, back then, we patient didn't know all the ins, outs, and options. Whatever the doctor said, we did.

There were visits from the lovely ladies of Reach To Recovery, bringing me books, prostheses, and other things. The one thing they said that stands out in my memory is, "Don't pick your cuticles and, above all, do not—DO NOT—ever let anyone draw blood from or give injections in your left arm." The best and soundest advice given by anyone!

You're probably wondering where I'm coming from—why I am talking about their warning. Hang in there, I'll get to it shortly. It's kind of hard keeping things in order—after all, it's been almost 23 years.

I made my post-op visits to the doctor, and he advised me not to drive for two or three weeks and not to play tennis for four weeks. Well, of course, I did not listen. I drove in ten days and played tennis in three weeks. Hey, I'm right handed, so I figured—why not?

On one of my visits to the doctor, they reminded me it was time for blood work to be done. I remember it was early in the morning, and since I had a big tennis match later in the day, I asked the doctor to draw the blood from my *left* arm. He said it would be no problem. That was the dumbest question I ever asked—and also the dumbest thing he's ever done. Here I must add that this was not my regular surgeon, but an internist who should have known better.

Prior to the above incident, I had some minor discomfort in the left arm, the mastectomy side, which was easily helped with just Tylenol or aspirin. Boy, did that change! About two weeks after the blood was drawn out of that arm, it began to swell—did it ever! It was now almost twice the size of my right arm. What to do? There was nothing I could do then except buy larger-sleeved clothing. I have adjusted to my arm over the years, but it has not always been easy. Different things, like the weather for one, make my arm ache. I just live with it.

I was fortunate enough to have a very positive outlook. In my mind, I rationalized that, "So what—

your breast is gone—but so is the cancer." I firmly believe that premise made my recovery much easier. In 1969, we were not privy to all the information we have now, and that may have helped me. You see, I really didn't know any better, so therefore, I just believed the cancer was gone and didn't worry about it. The lack of stress may have made my ability to get on with my life much easier.

By the way, I received no radiation or chemo-therapy. However, the surgeon did give me a shot. I have no idea what it was, because when I asked him, he said, "Don't worry about it. I give it to all my patients following your type of surgery."

If any of this has helped, I am happy. I am looking forward to 1994, please God, so I can celebrate 25 years. . .since my trip to the moon.

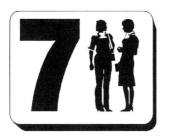 # THE DOCTOR-PATIENT RELATIONSHIP

I feel that people with cancer and their loved ones need to participate in their care and treatment. The diagnosis and treatment of cancer is so involved and complicated. You can play an important part in the treatment of cancer. It is your right and responsibility to use all the resources available in order to make your own choices and to live the richest, fullest life possible.

There are so many physicians, oncologists, radiologists, surgeons, anesthesiologists, and sometimes other specialists involved in cancer treatment. Physicians, especially cancer specialists, are busy people. Patients sometimes forget the questions they want to ask. My suggestion is to write down your questions ahead of time and take them with you to the doctor's office. You may also wish to take notes whenever talking with your doctor. You may want a family member to go along whenever you see the doctor. This person can help you remember what the doctor said.

The quality of information and the amount of time doctors and medical professionals spend with a patient can vary greatly. The kind of treatment you receive depends on how much your doctor knows about your specific cancer. You want your doctor to be very knowledgeable and to be able to communicate with you. However, you the patient must participate. You must be a partner with your medical team in the fight that will enable you to live your life in the way that is best for you. Your doctor should be someone for whom you have respect, and someone who sees you as a person, not just another patient.

Many women with breast cancer have a fear of being thought ignorant or pushy if they ask their doctors too many questions. It's OK to ask questions. What you are asking for is information. You are not attacking the treatment or the medical team giving you the treatment. You should not have a fear of taking up the doctor's valuable time. It's your body. It's your life. I think it is better to be a well-informed patient than to be a "good" patient. However, physicians are not mind readers. They need to know what the patient wants to know. It's up to you to take the first steps toward open communication with your doctors.

My advice is to ask, ask, and continue to ask questions you have. You are entitled to have your questions answered. If you aren't satisfied with your doctor's answers, find another doctor.

Of course, coping is an individual thing and what

works for one person may not work for another, but having a take charge attitude and being in control can make a difference. After all—you and your doctor have the same objective—*to get you well*.

Be considerate of your doctor's feelings. It is just as important to respect your doctor's view as it is for your doctor to respect your "view point." Most doctors are willing for the patient to help choose the course of treatment and to participate in the treatment plan. Family members should feel free to consult the physician and medical staff when they have questions and concerns. The doctor can advise them about their role in your treatment and how to handle problems.

Doctors need to appreciate what a scary time it is and that women have a sense of being in limbo after a diagnosis of breast cancer. Doctors need to realize that they are dealing with a person, not a breast. They need to take time to explain treatments and options, to answer questions, and to return patient's phone calls. Doctors need to listen to their patients.

Whenever there are tests, x–rays, or scans done on a patient, the doctor should be prompt in advising the patient of the results. It's very frustrating and scary to the already anxious patient to wait for days, not knowing the results of tests—while the test results are lying on a desk or in a basket in your doctor's office. The patient and doctor should have an understanding and an open line of communication.

Once you and your doctor have decided on your

course of treatment, you will feel more in control. You are better able to cope with your problems if you know what is being done for you, how it will be done, and what the prognosis may be.

Treatment may involve surgery, radiation therapy, and/or chemotherapy. These treatments may be used alone or in combination. Keep in mind that your physician is trained in the medical profession. He is responsible for determining your diagnosis and the way it is presented to you, including providing you with information about your treatment options. You are responsible for your choice in treatments.

Show an interest in your doctor as a person. Learn about his or her family, hobbies, and interests. Don't be afraid to hug your doctor, thank your doctor, and to let your doctor know you appreciate his efforts on your behalf. Be open with your health team. Tell them about your fears, your pain, and ask for whatever help you need.

According to the Memorial Sloan-Kettering Cancer Center, the best patient is the one who comes in with the attitude that she is willing to tolerate discomfort in an effort to get well. Your attitude plays a very important role. So you see, the responsibility for a harmonious relationship does not fall entirely on the doctor. It's also up to you to take steps toward communication. Remember, the members of your health team are all trying to help with your recovery. The key is teamwork!

For me, the best way to participate in my treatment was to be informed and to talk and share with my physicians. That meant taking time to read, research and ask many questions. Also, there were those medical professionals who did care, who were kind and considerate, and who took the time to listen to my fears and anxieties. They answered many questions for me. These medical professionals stand out in my mind, and to them I extend my gratitude. Their care contributed to my ability to fight to live.

A Patient's Bill Of Rights

1. You have the right to considerate and respectful care, and to participate actively in your health care.
2. You have the right to ask questions about your diagnosis, treatment, and prognosis—and to receive understandable answers.
3. You have the right to receive information necessary to give consent prior to treatment, and the right to say you don't understand and to have something clarified.
4. You have the right to refuse treatment and to get a second opinion.
5. You have the right to be heard and to be taken seriously.
6. You have the right to privacy and confidential-ity and to be treated with kindness by your health-care providers.
7. You have the right to ask about medications, treatment plans, side effects, and alternatives

before giving your approval or consent for anything.

8. You have the right to have telephone calls returned promptly and to know in advance what appointment times and what physicians are available.

9. You have the right to be told the truth if you ask about care and treatment plans.

10. You have the right to be fully informed as to the cost of your medical care and treatments, regardless of source of payment.

11. You have the right to communicate when something happens that you don't like, so that your doctor and you can find a productive way of dealing with each other.

12. You have the right to know what rules and regulations apply to you as a patient, and the right to change doctors if you are not satisfied with the care you are receiving.

--The American Cancer Society

RELATIONSHIPS

Family, Friends, and Public

Cancer—the word alone brings a flutter of fear and dread to the most courageous of hearts. When the disease strikes you or your loved one, your world suddenly shatters. You are devastated! You wonder how other people can seem so happy as if everything is normal. You feel the whole world should stop and share in your pain. This is the time you really need the love and support of your family and friends and those around you.

Living with cancer will be a little less difficult if everyone involved understands the effects of cancer and its treatments, and if everyone involved will discuss their concerns openly with each other.

Patient, family, and friends can expect periods of anxiety and depression. Sometimes, financial problems can be a real hardship due to loss of income and the high cost of treatments.

There are other problems, such as isolation from family and friends, physical problems, disruption of life goals, and an interrupted routine of normal activities.

Everyone affected must learn to make adjustments, and must never give up hope, but must try to work together so that daily life can be as rewarding as possible.

Everyone responds differently to cancer. At first, patient and family may refuse to accept the diagnosis. Many get so angry that they lash out at themselves, at other family members, or at the physicians. They may feel that fate has been unfair and unjust to them. The patient may fear the treatments, suffering pain, becoming dependent on others, and dying. They may want to give up.

Family members may feel helpless and unable to give support. They may feel guilty for not devoting enough time and energy to the patient. Children may feel responsible for a parent's illness.

Some of your friends, co-workers, and relatives may tend to fade away after your diagnosis of cancer. Some of them may just act differently toward you. They don't mean to do so; they are scared, too, or just don't know how to act or what to say. It may be that you are a threat to them by making them sense their own mortality. You must tell them to treat you just as they did before your diagnosis.

Other friends may step forward and be there for you. Whatever the case, you must strive to take charge.

Families and friends bear great emotional burdens and should be able to share them with each other and with you. By sharing, you and your family build a good foundation of mutual understanding and trust. This frees all of you to offer each other more love and support. It is so important not to shut each other out. You must work together so that life can be lived fully. Don't let your family detach themselves. Don't let your friends abandon you.

Being part of the family or a close friend doesn't mean you can make people talk about their feelings before they are ready to talk. However, sometimes listening or being a sounding board can be just as helpful as talking.

Each one of us learns to fill each day with the things that are important. You may help yourself by setting goals and making plans for the future. If you aren't making plans, you may subconsciously be giving up. If you can still do what you enjoyed before your diagnosis—start again. Regain as much control of your life as possible. The desire to recover from cancer and live can make a difference. A strong will to enjoy life can help a patient through rough periods and help them to get the most out of good periods.

It is important for everyone in your family support system to understand and realize that they can be most helpful if they can support your choices. However, they may simply not be able to grasp your point of view about life. There is no way for them to imagine something they have not dealt with and don't want to face. Their intentions may be good, but they are lacking in experience. It will, however, be helpful to you if your family members can look at the illness as a way to strengthen the family. Be a team— with family, friends, and loved ones.

For me, there were some family members who tried to detach themselves rather than feel the pain. I knew they cared very much for me, but they didn't seem to want to spend any time with me, especially if I were having a rough time after a treatment.

There were a few friends who wanted to run from me. It seemed when they learned I had a diagnosis of cancer, they stopped calling or coming to visit me. At first, I was rather upset about this, but I began to realize that my friends had to look at their own fear of death, and for them to accept that I was mortal meant that they were also mortal. There were some close friends who continued to be there for me during my surgeries, my treatments, and my recovery. These were not just fair weather friends; these were the real troopers who had been there for me during my husband's illness and death, and also during the illness and death of my mother.

Sometimes, the public can really send a cancer patient on a trip. Too often, people act as if cancer is contagious. On one occasion, I was shopping for a pair of walking shoes. This was shortly after my chemo treatments had ended and right after my second surgery. I was having trouble leaning forward to tie my shoes due to the recent surgery for breast cancer. I asked the shoe clerk if she would tie the shoes I was trying on. She was looking at me rather puzzled. I didn't look too great at the moment, as I had lost most of my hair and didn't have much sparkle in my eyes either. I told her I had recently had breast cancer surgery and now that I had completed some of my treatments, I wanted to try walking more each day. I told her I was purchasing these shoes for walking. She looked at me as if to say, "Why do you want walking shoes? You have cancer." She almost acted reluctant to assist me. She made me feel that she thought I was contagious and also as if to say she didn't feel like I would be doing much walking.

On another occasion, I was at the pharmacy to get a prescription filled. I saw an acquaintance of several years prior. We began talking. Upon learning that I had recently had breast cancer surgery she stated, "Well, you know it always comes back. Do you remember Rita? She had surgery for breast cancer and six months later the cancer came back and she is going to die."

I became numb. I didn't know how to respond. I wanted to yell at her to shut up. I wanted to cry. Needless to say, I did find the need to talk with my Life After Cancer counselor the following day.

It is just as important for family, relatives, and friends to know what not to say to a patient as it is to know what to say to one. I think people mean well. Sometimes they just don't think before talking.

Talking to Your Children

While you may be going through the worst emotional maelstrom of your life, your children are also going through tremendous readjustments. Let them know you're still there for them, although you might not be able to do all of the things you did before. Tell them you have had surgery, and that you will need to rest awhile. In the meantime, they can speed your recovery by helping you do some of the things you used to do for them.

Answer their questions openly and directly. Often children can imagine a scenario that is worse than the reality of the situation. Be alert to children who *do not* ask questions and seem withdrawn or hostile: know this is often their way of expressing worry and anxiety. Truthfully, they do care, but they need help in opening up and communicating with you. If you're having trouble communicating with children or other family members, ask your physician or a counselor at your local support group for help. Also, often support groups are available to help the children of those with cancer.

Remember, don't be afraid to burden your family. Most often, they are waiting and wanting to share with you, they just don't know how—or they're afraid of saying "the wrong thing." You may need to break the ice. When you do, you'll find most of your loved ones eager and ready to communicate with you.

 # STAR WARS, CHEMICAL WARFARE, TAKING YOUR MEDICATIONS

The percentage of women who will get breast cancer sometime during their lives is increasing. The American Cancer Society announced in January, 1991 that one of every nine women will have breast cancer during her lifetime. It also estimates that breast cancer will be diagnosed in about 180,000 women in 1992, and that in this same year, 46,000 women will die of the disease.

Researchers are not sure why more women are getting breast cancer. They believe it is partly due to increased emphasis on early detection. In the early 1980s, only about 15% of women had mammograms routinely, compared with 65% now.

Although having breast cancer remains one of the most frightening events in a woman's life, treatments have improved in recent years. Many women whose disease is in earlier stages can now have surgery to remove only the lump, followed by radiation therapy, instead of removing the entire breast.

Detection and Early Treatment

The fact that women *have* the option should encourage them to do monthly self-exams and to get routine mammograms. Every women should check herself every month and have a screening mammogram between the ages of 35 and 40, then one mammogram at least every two years under age 50, at which time women should have a yearly mammogram.

According to the American Cancer Society, women should look for a thickening or swelling of the breast, dimpling of the skin, scaliness, pain, or tenderness in the nipple. It is important that any woman who has a lump that can be felt have a biopsy to determine if it is cancerous. Although the mammogram is the most effective method for screening patients, it still misses about 10% of all lumps.

It is now standard practice for the physician, surgeon, radiation oncologist, medical oncologist, and patient to work together to plan and carry out each patient's treatment. If cancer is found on a biopsy, the patient may choose to have a *lumpectomy*.

A lumpectomy removes only the breast lump, along with a small margin of surrounding tissue. A *partial mastectomy* removes the lump, plus a wedge of normal tissue. The lumpectomy leaves only a small scar, and is usually followed up by radiation therapy. Not all women prefer lumpectomies. A lot of them feel more comfortable having a mastectomy. During surgery, doctors also remove a sample of

BREAST
SELF-EXAMINATION

Breast self-examination (BSE) should be done once a month so that you become familiar with the usual appearance and feel of your breasts. Familiarity makes it easier to notice any changes in the breast from one month to another. Early discovery of a change from what is "normal" is the main idea behind BSE. The outlook is much better if you detect cancer in an early stage.

If you menstruate, the best time to do BSE is 2 or 3 days after your period ends, when your breasts are least likely to be tender or swollen. If you no longer menstruate, pick a particular day, such as the first day of the month, to remind yourself it is time to do BSE.

Here is one way to do BSE:

1. Stand before a mirror. Inspect both breasts for anything unusual such as any discharge from the nipples or puckering, dimpling, or scaling of the skin.

The next two steps are designed to emphasize any change in the shape or contour of your breasts. As you do them, you should be able to feel your chest muscles tighten.

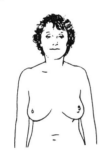

2. Watching closely in the mirror, clasp your hands behind your head and press your hands forward.

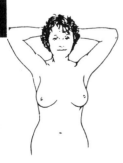

3. Next, press your hands firmly on your hips and bow slightly toward your mirror as you pull your shoulders and elbows forward.

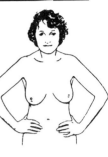

Some women do the next part of the exam in the shower because fingers glide over soapy skin, making it easy to concentrate on the texture underneath.

4. Raise your left arm. Use three or four fingers of your right hand to explore your left breast firmly, carefully, and thoroughly. Beginning at the outer edge, press the flat part of your fingers in small circles, moving the circles slowly around the breast. Gradually work toward the nipple. Be sure to cover the entire breast. Pay special attention to

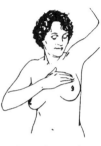

the area between the breast and the underarm, including the underarm itself. Feel for any unusual lump or mass under the skin.

5. Gently squeeze the nipple and look for a discharge. (If you have any discharge during the month— whether or not it is during BSE— see your doctor.) Repeat steps 4 and 5 on your right breast.

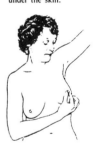

6. Steps 4 and 5 should be repeated lying down. Lie flat on your back with your left arm over your head and a pillow or folded towel under your left shoulder. This position flattens the breast and makes it easier to examine. Use the same circular motion described earlier. Repeat the exam on your right breast.

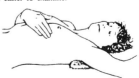

From a publication of the National Cancer Institute. Reprints of the pamphlet, "Breast Exams: What You Should Know," can be obtained by calling 1-800-4-CANCER.

lymph nodes from the woman's armpit to see if they show any evidence of cancer. It is now recognized that axillary lymph nodes are not an effective barrier to tumor spread. However, they can provide information about the risk of recurrence and metastasis and the need for adjuvant therapy. Doctors look at several other factors to predict who will have a recurrence, including the size of the tumor, the amount of DNA in the cells that may activate normal cells to turn cancerous, and the presence of an enzyme that is thought to be made by cancer cells.

Pathologists also look to see if the tumor has estrogen and progesterone *receptors*—proteins that bind with the hormones and support the growth of the tumor. Women who have the positive receptors are usually given the anti-estrogen drug, tamoxifen, which keeps the cancer cells from getting the hormones they need to grow. Women whose lymph nodes test positive usually get chemotherapy treatments.

Radiation

Radiation treatments can be effective in any stage of breast cancer. The treatments are usually given for six weeks. Sometimes, radiation alone can destroy a tumor that can't be removed surgically. It is more often used after a lumpectomy. Sometimes, radiation is used after a mastectomy, especially if the cancer is in the surrounding skin and breast tissue. The most common side effect of radiation is fatigue.

The treatments can also thicken breast tissue and darken skin. More emphasis is now placed on focusing on the site to be radiated, while minimizing damage to surrounding healthy tissue.

Chemotherapy

After radiation, chemotherapy is the most common post-surgical treatment for breast cancer.

Different drugs, administered in combination, are available today. Doctors usually start out with the maximum dosage recommended for a patient's body mass, then fine-tune the treatments to relieve any toxic side effects. Because the drugs are meant to be toxic, they can wreak havoc on healthy cells.

Nausea and vomiting can result when the drugs trigger areas of the brain that control nausea. Only about twenty percent of the women receiving the most widely prescribed chemotherapy combination—known as *CMF*, for Cytoxan, methotrexate, and 5-fluorouracil—report nausea and vomiting. Patients receiving the *CAF* combination, which contains the powerful drug adriamycin instead of methotrexate, tend to suffer more serious discomfort. Some doctors choose to prescribe the more toxic CAF in advanced stages of cancer because is slightly more effective in shrinking tumors quickly.

One of the most valuable developments in cancer care, available as of February, 1991, is the drug *Zofran*. It relieves more instances of queasy stomach, that other drugs cannot help. Zofran appears to have no major side effects. It is currently administered in two or three daily intravenous doses.

For many breast cancer patients, the more traumatic side effect of chemotherapy is hair loss. This can occur anywhere. Patients who go bald may have a different texture of hair when it returns. While the adriamycin in CAF chemotherapy virtually always causes hair loss soon after treatment begins, milder CMF combinations only cause complete baldness in ten to fifteen percent of patients.

A more complicated consequence of chemotherapy is low white blood cell count—which makes a person more susceptible to infection. Probably the most common side effect of chemo is fatigue, loss of appetite, unusual food cravings, weight loss, weight gain, fluid retention, diarrhea, constipation, mouth sores, and susceptibility to infection. However, please remember that for each of these side effects, your doctor can prescribe medication to lessen the adverse effects.

Hormone Therapies

Hormone therapies block the growth of cancer cells that depend on estrogen and progesterone. These treatments often last indefinitely, unless the cancer returns or a patient develops an intolerance to the drug. *Tamoxifen*, the most common anti-estrogen hormone treatment, comes in pill form under the commercial name of *Nolvadex*. Hormone therapies can cause hot flashes, nausea, and irregular periods.

About three to five percent of the women who take tamoxifen develop blood clots.

Bone marrow transplants and, more recently, stem cell transplants are rapidly becoming more important in cancer treatments. Only in the past twenty years has medical knowledge advanced to the point where these techniques could be developed. These techniques involve intravenous administration of immature blood cells capable of reproducing themselves and repopulating empty bone marrow.

Alternative Treatments

Alternative treatments include therapies involving diets, vitamins, use of herbs, mental techniques, laughter, psychic healing, acupuncture, biofeedback, and others, which some patients may choose instead of the conventional or traditional treatments. There are alternatives, such as certain beverages to drink, pastes to rub on the skin, magnetic forces to direct at various parts of the body, potions made from natural or chemical substances, and detoxification.

While I prefer to use any available therapies in addition to, and not instead of, conventional or traditional therapies, I feel this is a highly personal decision, and a choice that a patient can make. Surgery, radiation, chemotherapy, and hormonal therapy have been the accepted cancer treatments for a long time.

Probably what sustains breast cancer patients with their treatments is the notion that their current

how bad they feel," says Larry Norton, M.D., of New York's Memorial Sloan-Kettering Cancer Center, "their cancer cells feel worse."

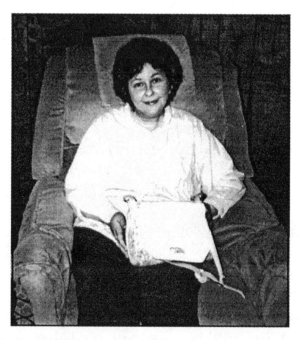

Painful Therapy: Norma Suzette in 1989. "After surgery, chemo, and radiation, I weighed 200 pounds. My arm was so swollen, I couldn't button the sleeve of my blouse, and my grand daughter wore my wig (to play dress-up) more than I did. The good news is, I did lose the extra 50 pounds within two years!"

Tamoxifen (Oral)*

A commonly used brand name is *Nolvadex*.

About The Medicine

Tamoxifen (ta-MOX-i-fen) is a medicine that blocks the effects of the hormone estrogen in the body. It is used to treat some cases of breast cancer in women. If any of the following information causes you special concern, or if you want more information about this medicine and its use, check with your doctor, nurse, or pharmacist. Remember, keep this and all other medicines out of the reach of children and never share your medicines with others.

Before Using This Medicine

Discuss with your doctor the possible side effects that may be caused by this medicine. Some of them may be serious and/or long term.

Tell your doctor, nurse, and pharmacist if you:
- Are allergic to any medicine, either prescription or nonprescription.
- Are pregnant or intend to become pregnant while using this medicine.
- Are breast-feeding an infant.
- Currently take any other prescription or non-prescription medicine.
- Have any other medical problems.

Proper Use of This Medicine

Use this medicine only as directed by your doctor. Do not use more or less of it, and do not use it more often than your doctor ordered.

Tamoxifen commonly causes nausea and vomiting. However, it is very important that you continue to use the medicine, even if you begin to feel ill. Ask your doctor, nurse, or pharmacist for ways to lessen these effects.

If you vomit shortly after taking a dose of tamoxifen, check with your doctor.

If you miss a dose of this medicine, do not take the missed dose at all and do not double the next one. Instead, go back to your regular dosing schedule and check with your doctor.

Precautions While Using This Medicine

It is very important that your doctor check your progress at regular visits to make sure this medicine is working properly and to check for unwanted effects.

Tamoxifen may make you more fertile. It is best to use some type of birth control while you are taking it. However, do not use oral contraceptives (the Pill), since they may change the effects of tamoxifen. Tell your doctor right away if you think you have become pregnant while taking this medicine.

Side Effects of This Medicine

Side Effects That Should Be Reported As

Soon As Possible:
- Blurred vision
- Pain or swelling in legs
- Confusion
- Shortness of breath
- Weakness or sleepiness

Side Effects That Usually Do Not Require Medical Attention:

These possible side effects may go away during treatment; however, if they continue, or are bothersome, check with your doctor, nurse, or pharmacist.
- Bone pain
- Changes in periods
- Headaches
- Hot flashes
- Itching in genital area
- Nausea or vomiting
- Skin rash or dryness
- Vaginal bleeding or discharge
- Weight gain

Other side effects not listed above may also occur in some patients. If you notice any other effects, check with your doctor, nurse, or pharmacist.

Reprints of this Tamoxifen Bulletin, plus a lot of other information about cancer and its treatments, are available through the Cancer Information Service hotline: 1-800-4-CANCER.

Follow-up After Breast Cancer Treatment

After your diagnosis of breast cancer and the treatment option that you and your physician choose, your treatment plan does not stop with the surgery and completion of chemotherapy, radiation, and hormonal treatment. You will need careful follow-up treatment and monitoring by your physician, surgeon, and oncologist. Good follow-up care is necessary for several reasons, among these, to monitor the response to treatments and to detect any recurrence.

The standard follow-up care involves regular physical examinations and mammograms. Usually, the doctor will check you every three to four months for the first two years, and every six months after that. Your surgeon will follow you at regular intervals. You will be followed by your medical oncologist and your radiation oncologist. Other tests and scans include the following: Blood chemistry profiles (liver and kidneys), tumor markers (CEA, bone, CA 15-3), imaging studies—abdominal—(CT, MRI, radioisotope scans, and x-rays) to look for metastasis, bone scans, chest x-rays, and x-rays of any positive areas on bone scan, and any special studies deemed necessary for questionable area.

With some cancers we can be reasonably sure that if they have not returned within a few years, they won't. However, breast cancer is not one of them. It's usually a slow growing cancer, and there are people who have reoccurrences ten or even twenty years later after the original diagnosis. Breast cancer is really a chronic disease. Don't expect a recurrence, but be prepared for it.

You need information to carry out your role in managing your health care. Keep accurate, up-to-date records of the medical care you receive for cancer and any other illnesses. Keep track of your check-up schedule and your medical history, the tests, the scans, and the medications. You will want to take the health steps your doctor recommends.

Long–term health needs for cancer survivors vary from person to person. As you face forward, be kind to yourself. Don't be afraid to say *no*. Take time for the activities that you enjoy, taking one thing at a time. Set your priorities. Don't try to be "superwoman." Try to stay focused on the positive.

Women at High Risk for Getting Breast Cancer

- Women at age 50 and over
- Women whose mother or sister has had breast cancer
- Women who have already had breast cancer in one breast
- Women with precancerous breast disease
- Women with breast cysts proven by aspiration or surgery
- Women who have not had any children

- Women who had their first child after 30
- Women who began menstruating at age 12 or younger
- Women who experience menopause after 55
- Women who are obese

Symptoms of Breast Cancer

- Lump or thickening of the breast
- Discharge from the nipple
- Dimpling or puckering of the skin
- Retraction of the nipple
- Scaly skin around the nipple
- Other changes in skin color, texture, such as "orange peel" skin
- Swelling, redness, or feeling of heat in the breast
- Lumps under the arm

Staging of Breast Cancer

The staging of cancer has several purposes. It is a useful way of identifying the extent of the cancer—its size, degree of growth, and spread. It provides an estimate of the prognosis, and also provides a common set of criteria against which doctors can compare treatments for a specific type and stage of cancer. In the commonly used TNM System, T stands for the size of the tumor, N for the degree of spread to lymph nodes, and M for the presence of metastasis. TO means the tumor was completely removed by the biopsy. *T1* indicates the smallest tumor; *T2*, *T3*, and *T4* indicate larger tumors that may have grown into surrounding tissues. *NO* means that nearby lymph nodes are free of cancer. *N1*, *N2*, and *N3* signify increasing node involvement. *MO* means that no distant metastases have been found.

You must refer to the TNM Chart for each cancer to be sure of the specific stage.

T = Primary Tumor
N = Regional lymph nodes
M = Distant metastasis

Primary Tumor(T)

TO	No evidence of primary tumor
TIS	Carcinoma in situ; intraductal carcinoma, lobular carcinoma in situ, or Paget's disease of the nipple with no tumor
T2	Tumor more than 2 cm. but not more than 5 cm. in greatest dimension
T3	Tumor more than 5 cm. in greatest dimension
T4	Tumor of any size with direct extension to chest wall or skin or surrounding breast tissue

Regional Lymph Nodes (N) (Clinical)

NO	No regional lymph node metastasis
Nl	Metastasis to movable axillary lymph

	nodes
N2	Metastasis to axillary lymph nodes fixed to one another
N3	Metastasis to internal mammary lymph nodes.

Distant Metastasis (M)

MX	Presence of distant metastasis cannot be assessed
MO	No distant metastasis
M1	Distant metastasis

Stage Grouping

STAGE O	Tis	NO	MO
STAGE I	T1	NO	MO
STAGE IIA	TO	N1	MO
	T1	N1	MO
	T2	NO	MO
STAGE IIB	T2	N1	MO
	T3	NO	MO
STAGE IIIA	TO	N2	MO
	T1	N2	MO
	T2	N2	MO
	T3	Nl, N2	MO
STAGE IIIB	T4	Any N	MO
	Any T	N3	MO
STAGE IV	Any T	Any N	M1

Prosthesis or Reconstructive Surgery?

After breast cancer surgery, you have the option of wearing a prosthesis or having reconstructive surgery. The chances are that you made that decision prior to your surgery. Sometimes, reconstruction is done at the time of the mastectomy. The important thing is that you have the choice of making the decision that is right for you.

After having a mastectomy, there are medical reasons why you should wear a prosthesis form to replace the missing breast. The weight of the remaining breast can cause shoulder, neck, and back pain. Also, you should plan to buy a prosthesis for your own emotional well being. It can mean a difference in your recovery. The proper fit can give you a cheerful feeling of well being.

There are several places to buy a prosthesis: department stores, special outlets, surgical supply houses, or by mail order.

Some patients wear a prosthesis only a few hours a day, while others sleep with a prosthesis on. Most doctors will tell you to wait until the scar is fully healed before getting fitted for a breast prosthesis. However, soft forms can be worn from the very beginning.

Whenever you shop for a prosthesis, it is a good idea to take someone with you. Make sure you try on several kinds and be sure the one you finally buy is what you really want. There are many different breast forms on the market. Make sure you shop around. It is a good idea to wear figure revealing clothes when you are trying on a prosthesis. It is important to pay close attention to how it feels and how it fits. The form should match your other breast from the side, the bottom and the front.

There are different kinds of prostheses available. There are the silicone gel-filled form, the liquid or air-filled form, the foam rubber form and a lightweight polyester form. Ask the American Cancer Society or a Reach to Recovery volunteer for a list of prosthesis options. Usually a prosthesis is flesh-colored and sized to match the remaining breast. The flat side goes against the wall of the chest area and the tail goes toward the arm pit.

Most insurance companies will cover at least a part of the cost of the first prosthesis. The doctor must write a prescription for the form.

You may have chosen to have breast reconstruction. If so, it is a good idea to ask your surgeon for a consultation with a plastic surgeon before your mastectomy.

The results and difficulties with reconstruction will vary with each individual. Most patients are very pleased with the results of reconstruction. They say it makes them feel more like themselves.

There are different types of surgery performed for breast reconstruction. A board-certified plastic surgeon should do the breast reconstruction. Ask your doctor to recommend someone for a consultation or call a teaching hospital. You may wish to talk with someone who has had reconstructive breast surgery.

Whatever your choice may be, just be sure you feel good about your decision.

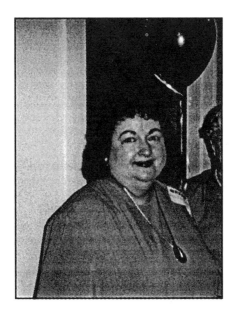

Co-author, Allie Fair, at a Life After Cancer-Pathways "Survivor's Day" celebration in 1992. She says, "I'm glad that ladies have a choice whether to have reconstructive surgery or to wear a prosthesis. Just feel good about your decision and know that it is OK to change your mind."

The Cancer Conqueror's Ten Key Beliefs

I believe. . .
1. I am in charge of my cancer, my cancer is not in charge of me.
2. Cancer is a reversible disease.
3. My treatment is effective and has minimal side-effects.
4. My immune system is powerful and can effectively inhibit cancerous growth.
5. My body, and thus my immune system, is affected by my mind and by my spirit.
6. My mind and my spirit are affected by my emotions.
7. Cancer is a message to change.
8. The key lesson is that peace of mind is the goal.
9. Genuine peace comes from understanding there is a God who knows me and loves me. And God loves me even though God knows me.
10. I believe I become a cancer conqueror not because I go into remission, but because I am a new person.

—*from* Possibilities, *March/April 1989*

10 SEA SHELLS, SHAMROCKS, AND TIGER LILIES

Lessons From Our Lives

Laughter! What a marvelous thing. It can be experienced doing the most unusual things. Take, for instance, an event that happened when three friends (who were all breast cancer survivors) were at the beach together.

They were getting ready for bed, when one of them said she had to wash her prosthesis. The other two decided they would wash theirs, too, even though they didn't think they really needed washing, since they were told it extended the life of the "boob." Not many people can imagine what a sight it was as each woman took her prosthesis to the sink, washed it with Ivory soap (which is 99.44% pure), rinsed it, and then patted it dry with a towel.

They laughed about the differences in size and then laughed more as they expressed the collective opinion that most people would think they were crazy if they were witnessing this scene.

--nsj

A special breast cancer survivor we know told us that after her third chemotherapy treatment, her hair began to fall out rather quickly. As it was falling out, she had her daughter hook up the extension hose of the vacuum cleaner and vacuum her head and clothes so the hair wouldn't float around everywhere.

--nsj

There was a breast cancer survivor who was an excellent seamstress. After her mastectomy, she had begun the habit of using her lightweight foam prosthesis (when wearing it) as a handy pin cushion while sewing. One day, she answered a knock at her front door and gave the person standing there quite a shock! Noticing how the visitor's eyes were riveted on her chest, she looked down at herself and quickly tried to explain the situation.

--nsj

Upon seeing you for the first time after your mastectomy, (and if you are wearing a prosthesis) lots of people will stare at your chest—trying to figure out which one is your real breast and which one is the fake. When you notice this happening, you could just smile and say, "Only my surgeon knows for sure."

--nsj

That's Entertainment!

Humor really is one of our best "medicines." Why

not treat yourself today to some of the following funny books, audio cassettes, and movies? This selection comes courtesy of the Comprehensive Cancer Center at Duke University:

BOOKS

Title	Author
Without Feathers	Woody Allen
The Rescue of Miss Yaskell and Other Pipe Dreams	Russell Baker
Murphy's Law	Arthur Bloch
Crackers	Roy Blount, Jr.
The Grass is Always Greener Over the Septic Tank	Erma Bombeck
Chocolate: The Consuming Passion	Sandra Boynton
I Never Danced at the White House	Art Buchwald
Dr. Burns' Prescription for Happiness	George Burns
Oh Heavenly Dog!	Joe Camp
Decline and Fall of Practically Everybody	Will Cuppy
The Fourth Garfield Treasury	Jim Davis
The Complete Mother	Phyllis Diller
Dictionary for Yankees	Bill Dwyer
How to Eat Like a Child: And Other Lessons in Not Being a Grown-Up	Delia Ephron
Is it Friday Yet, Luann?	Greg Evans
I Never Met a Kid I Liked	W.C. Fields
Heathcliff: Smooth Sailing	George Gately

How to Make Yourself Miserable	Dan Greenburg
Shoot Low, Boys—They're Ridin' Shetland Ponies	Lewis Grizzard
The Blarney Stone American West	John Hewlett
Happy to Be Here	Garrison Keillor
Please Don't Eat the Daisies	Jean Kerr
The Far Side Gallery Two	Gary Larson
The Greatest Shoe on Earth	Jeff MacNelly
The Great Wall Street Joke Book	John Pizzuto
The Reagan Chronicles	Dwane Powell
Rally Round the Flag, Boys!	Max Schulman
Welcome to the Real World	Wes Smith
It's Hard to Be Hip Over Thirty and Other Tragedies of Married Life	Judith Viorst
You All Spoken Here	Roy Wilder, Jr.
Mouse Breath Conformity and Other Social Ills	Jonathan Winters

AUDIO CASSETTES

Title	**Performer**
Bloopers	Anonymous
The Ambassador of Goodwill	Jerry Clower
Live in Picayune	Jerry Clower
Top Gum	Jerry Clower
The Best of Bill Cosby	Bill Cosby
Is a Very Funny Fellow, Right!	Bill Cosby
Wonderfulness	Bill Cosby
200 M.P.H.	Bill Cosby
I Don't Get No Respect	Rodney Dangerfield
The Best of W.C. Fields	W.C. Fields
All the President's Wits	Gerald Gardner
The Works	Groucho Marx

News from Lake Wobegon—Summer	Garrison Keillor
News from Lake Wobegon—Winter	Garrison Keillor
Ogden Nash Reads	Ogden Nash
What Becomes a Semi-legend Most?	Joan Rivers
Crackin' Up	Ray Stevens
Surely You Joust	Ray Stevens
He Thinks He's Ray Stevens	Ray Stevens

VIDEOCASSETTES
Humor/Comedy
Airplane!
All of Me
Blazing Saddles
Making Mr. Right
Privates on Parade
The Return of the Pink Panther
Some Like It Hot
The Making of the Stooges
The Films of Laurel and Hardy
Volunteers

Science Fiction
Star Wars
Star Trek IV: The Voyage Home
Back to the Future

Adventures
Cool Hand Luke
Crocodile Dundee
High Road to China
Silverado

Romancing the Stone
Jewel of the Nile
Patton
Raiders of the Lost Arc
Silverado
Superman
Top Gun

Reflections

After your mastectomy or lumpectomy, when the incision is still very tender, wear a shirt with two pockets and stuff Kleenex in the appropriate pocket to even out the look. This is a comfortable way to heal and make a good appearance at the same time if you are fairly small busted.

--nsj

After a mastectomy, lumpectomy, or biopsy, moving your arm is very important as it helps prevent the forming of adhesions (scar tissue) which could later limit the full movement of your arm.

--nsj

If you don't know what to say to a woman about her mastectomy, radiation, chemotherapy, other treatments, or emotional distress—try something simple like "I'm sorry you are suffering right now." Kind, sincere words are so appreciated during such rough times.

--nsj

The idea of relaxation leads naturally into the subject of rest and sleep. Before you had breast cancer, you may not have thought of resting during the day. And sleep was something you did only when everything you needed or wanted to do was finished. Now, you might consider revising your life style.

If you use all your energy and don't get adequate rest, your body won't have anything left over for the immune system. The major organs, such as the brain, lungs, and heart, get their share first—the immune system is last. Consequently, it gets fed best while the other organs are at rest.

Taking out a few minutes to rest several times during the day does wonders for the immune system.

--rmc

I've heard the old saying "you gotta have heart" and never really knew what it meant. After all of the trauma I have personally experienced fighting breast cancer, I now know what it means. After watching some of the other patients who sat with me in many waiting rooms, I began to realize what it meant to "have heart." We were all in the same boat as we waited for a nurse to call us back for treatments that were painful, sickening, and sometimes frightening.

There were days when I went for my treatments without enough intestinal fortitude to carry me through it. Most of the time, I had to look deep inside myself to find a spark of courage and fan it to life. Occasionally, though, another cancer patient, nurse, doctor, friend, or family member would loan me enough "heart" to continue on. Everyone needs a pat on the back, a kind word, or to borrow a little bit of "heart" from someone occasionally. I was always happy to lend it to somebody on the days I had extra.

--nsj

I don't know how much longer I will live—none of us do. But I do know that I'm going to *live* each day to the fullest. I will die on only one day of my life—the last—that's all that's required of me, and I don't intend to waste my remaining days anticipating that day. There are too many wonderful things to accomplish. Each day is a gift and I intend to treasure all of them.

--rmc

If we wait until we become perfect before we love ourselves—we will waste our lives.

--Louise Hay

Sometimes, people seem like shooting stars through each others lives. Take for example, what happened to three members of a support group who took a trip to the beach just for the fun of it. They were playing bingo one night and started talking to a woman sitting at their table. They discovered that she was also a breast cancer survivor (ten years) and that she made a two hour trip to play bingo nearly every week. She explained that after she recovered from her treatments she decided she would take the time to do things she enjoyed and that was why she was there playing bingo.

It's important to do something you enjoy every day, simply because it gives you happiness. It doesn't have to be anything big or unusual—just something special to you that makes you feel good.

--nsj

The presence of cancer is a reminder that we are mortal. We have limited time and don't have moments to waste on "I should haves" and "what ifs." We must concentrate on each moment. Therefore, we must cherish each day of our lives. We must hug and be hugged. We must stop to smell the flowers, to notice the dew on a rose petal, or to catch a glimpse of a rainbow. We must make our time count.

--afs

About two days after my diagnosis of breast cancer, I found the sunrise so beautiful that I sat through a traffic light enjoying the view—until the person in the car behind me began honking their horn. I didn't get angry with him and I hoped he wasn't angry with me. I just drove on through the green light and continued to enjoy the beautiful sunlight of another day in my life.

--afs

Victory over cancer does not depend on living a normal life span. Victory is living each moment of your life fully.

--afs

Christmas 1989—from my couch I saw Christmas through the eyes of a child once more.

--afs

Autumn of 1990. My street is quiet; I am alone. I stand gazing out the bedroom window with tears streaming down my cheeks. The question before me is "What now, Lord?" I am a person geared for productivity. I have just resigned from a job I did for the past twelve years—due to my multiple health problems. I have been fighting so hard for my life this past year.

Most members of my family live in other towns. Some family members I haven't heard from in months. I feel so alone and scared. It seems that there are so many mountains to climb, and so many valleys to pass through. My disability has not been approved and my financial problems are taxing on my low energy. There are tests, scans, x-rays, and other procedures to be done on my tired body. Can I trust the mammography equipment this time? Do I dare hope for tomorrow? Several Scripture verses come to my mind: "God is my refuge and my strength—a very present help in trouble," "Cast all your care on Him for He cares for you," and "My strength is made perfect in weakness."

I think about the birds of the air, the flowers, the lilies of the field. . .I see two squirrels chasing each other and I smile. I am going to walk unafraid. I will not waste one more precious minute of this lovely day. I will look for the beauty in this day and enjoy its sunshine or its rain. The falling leaves are so colorful. This is the day the Lord has made and I will be thankful for it. I am at peace with myself.

--afs

For me, my religious faith learned as a child in my little mountain home was a source of strength. I found solace and strength in reading certain passages from my Bible. For example: "What time I am afraid, I will trust in Thee" (Psalm 56:3), "Be strong and of a good courage, fear not, nor be afraid, neither be thou dismayed; for the Lord thy God is with thee whithersoever thou goest" (Joshua 1:9), and "Beloved, I wish above all things that thou mayest prosper and be in health, even as thy soul prospereth" (3 John 2). I also found much comfort in listening to some of the old time hymns.

During my cancer experience and journey toward healing, the scriptures held special meaning for me.

--afs

I'm getting more out of each day than I used to get out of a week. We are never the same after cancer as we were before and now living one day at a time brings me peace, joy, and serenity. I love and accept myself just the way I am and, as the saying goes, " I am the master of my fate and the captain of my soul." I can see the sun coming over the horizon and I feel blessed.

--afs

Believe that life is worth living and your belief will help create the fact.

--William James

I shut the door on yesterday and threw the key away. Tomorrow has no fears for me since I have found today.

--Unknown

Yesterday is a canceled check. Tomorrow is a promissory note. Today is ready cash—spend it.

--Unknown

What the caterpillar calls the end of the world— the Master calls a butterfly.

--Richard Bach

The best rose bush after all, is not that which has the fewest thorns, but that which bears the finest roses.

--Henry Van Dyke

Daydreams are. . .
Swirling, sparkling, dancing clouds of dreams.
Shining, softly floating on sunbeams.
Mint green, pale pink peach, and baby blue.
Mingled, interwoven thoughts both old and new.
Skipping, darting, flashing through the mind.
Smiling! Creating images to pass the time.

--nsj

Reflections. . .
On a recent visit back to my hometown, I was reflecting on memories. Most of them were pleasant—the smell of popcorn on the stove, the smell of gingerbread cooking, the crackle of fire in the fireplace, the feeling of being wrapped in a fluffy soft blanket, the sound of the babbling stream, the sounds of nature. I have decided that when the stresses and forces in my life begin to overpower me, I will slip back to that time and place in childhood where there was warmth, where there was security, and where there was love. I will do something that reminds me of that special time and those warm feelings. I will savor those feelings, and then I will know that I have the courage to continue my journey.

—afs

Recommended Reading

Affirmations, Meditations, and Encouragements for Women Living with Breast Cancer, by Linda Dackman, Lowell House Publishers, 1991. An inspirational, uplifting book. A resource to strengthen those women with breast cancer from diagnosis through treatment and to recovery.

Choices: Realistic Alternatives in Cancer Treatment, by Marion Morra and Eve Potts, Avon, 1987. This book has many questions and answers about all kinds of cancer and cancer treatments. A helpful book for cancer patients at the time of diagnosis.

Dr. Susan Love's Breast Book, by Susan M. Love, M.D., with Karen Lindsey, Addison Wesley, Menlo Park, California, 1990. Dr. Love, a breast surgeon, discusses all conditions of the breast and breast cancer treatments. A good reference book for patients recovering from cancer.

First You Cry, by Betty Rollins, New American Library, New York, 1976. This book is by a well known TV broadcaster who wrote one of the first books on a woman's personal experience with breast cancer. The book was later made into a movie.

Hanging in There: Living Well on Borrowed Time, by Natalie Davis Spingarn, Stein and Day, Briarcliff Manor, New York, 1982. A journalist writes of her personal experience with breast cancer and the major issues facing people with serious illnesses.

Heart Thoughts, by Louise L. Hay, Hay House, Inc., 1990. Louise L. Hay shares her philosophies and wisdom for daily living in meditations and affirmations.

Life Wish, by Jill Ireland, Little, Brown, Boston,

1987. The actress writes of her personal battle with breast cancer.

Love, Medicine, and Miracles, by Bernie S. Siegel, M.D., Harper and Row Publishers, New York, 1986. Relates lessons learned about self-healing. Based on a surgeon's experience with exceptional patients.

Peace, Love, and Healing, by Bernie S. Siegel, M.D., Harper and Row Publishers, New York, 1989. By the author of *Love, Medicine, and Miracles*, this book illustrates how our mind influences the body and explores the role of self-healing.

Man to Man: When the Woman You Love Has Breast Cancer, by Andy Murcia and Bob Stewart, St. Martin's Press, New York, 1989. A resource book by two men about breast cancer; for men and the women they love. In the same week, they learned that their wives, actress Ann Jillian and housewife Martha Stewart, had breast cancer. They address the impact of their wives' breast cancer on them.

Moms Don't Get Sick, by Pat Brack with Ben Brack, Melius Publishing Corporation, 1990. This writer deals primarily with her relationship with her ten year–old son, Ben, after her diagnosis of breast cancer. A helpful book for women with young children.

No Less a Woman, by Deborah H. Hahane, M.S.W., Prentice Hall Press, 1990. A writer and health educator, as well as a breast cancer survivor, writes about her own experiences with the disease and the personal stories of ten women she interviewed.

Of Tears and Triumphs, by Georgia and Bud Photopulus, Congdon and Weed, New York, 1988. A couple writes about dealing with Georgia's cancer crisis over a 20 year period.

Questions and Answers About Pain Control: A Guide for People with Cancer and Their Families, American Cancer Society, 1986. Discusses pain control using both medical and nonmedical methods. Emphasizes explanation, self-help, and participation.

Reach to Recovery: After Mastectomy, The American Cancer Society. A patient guide with helpful information and "how-to's" for a woman who has had a mastectomy.

Sexuality and Cancer: For the Woman Who Has Cancer and Her Partner, American Cancer Society, 1988. Gives information about this area of concern to the patient and her partner. Includes a resource list.

Spinning Straw Into Gold: Your Emotional Recovery From Breast Cancer, by Ronnie Kaye, M.F.C.C., Fireside/Simon and Schuster, Inc., 1991. A psychotherapist shares her personal experience about breast cancer and also the stories of her clients. It is a comprehensive guide to emotional recovery from breast cancer.

Surviving Cancer, by Danette G. Kauffman, Acropolis Books, 1989. A practical guide to experiencing cancer and its treatment, with an emphasis on lists of resources for managing the medical, emotional, and financial aspects of the disease.

Taking Time: Support for People With Cancer and the People Who Care About Them, National Cancer Institute, 1988. A sensitively written booklet for people with cancer and their families. It addresses feelings and concerns of others in similar situations and how they have coped.

Talking With Your Doctor, American Cancer Society, 1987. This book has numerous suggestions for effective doctor/patient communication.

The Cancer Conqueror: An Incredible Journey to Wellness, by Greg Anderson, Andrews and McMeel, Kansas City, 1990. This is the story of how he and his family played a role in his recovery—after his doctor told him he had thirty days to live and sent him home. A book about positive living.

The Healing Journey, by O. Carl Simonton, M.D., Bantam Books, 1992. In this sequel to *Getting Well Again*, an extraordinary doctor and one of his patients offer healing ideas to anyone with a life threatening illness.

Triumph: Getting Back to Normal When You Have Cancer, by Marion Morra and Eve Potts, Avon, 1990. The authors of *Choices* write another question–and–answer book for cancer survivors.

Women Talk About Breast Surgery, by Amy Gross and Dee Ito, Clarkson Potter Publishers, 1990. A collection of stories and conversations with women who have had breast surgery (biopsy, lumpectomy, mastectomy, and reconstructive surgery).

The Woman's Book of Courage, by Susan Patton Thoele, Conari Press, 1991. An inspirational book of reflections and affirmations. For women in transition or recovery—and anyone who wishes to enhance their personal power.

APPENDIX A

Where to Get More Information

For more information about breast cancer and its treatments, certified centers that do early detection screening, or for a referral to a support group in your area, contact:

1-800-4-CANCER   Cancer Information Service
Duke Comprehensive Cancer
Center
Erwin Square, Suite 10
2020 W. Main Street
Durham, NC 27705

1-800-ACS-2345   American Cancer Society
90 Park Avenue
New York, NY 10016

1-608-263-2118   Cancer Prevention Program
Wisconsin Tamoxifen Study
1300 University Avenue, 7C
Madison, WI 53706

1-800-541-3259   National Lymphedema
Network

2211 Post Street, Suite 404
San Francisco, CA 94115

1-404-320-3333   Reach To Recovery, ACS
Tower Place
3340 Peachtree Road, NE
Atlanta, GA 30026

1-800-221-2141   National Breast Cancer Organization (Y-ME)
18220 Harwood Avenue
Homewood, IL 60430

1-212-719-0154   National Alliance of Breast
Cancer Organizations
(NABCO)
1180 Avenue of the Americas,
Second Floor
New York, NY 10036

1-505-764-9956   National Coalition for Cancer
Survivorship (NCCS)
323 Eighth Street, SW
Albuquerque, NM 87102

APPENDIX B

Contemplating the Future: Norma

The future. What do I want to say about the future? Well, first of all, I'm so glad I have one. I have more time in the future because of medical technology, scientists, new knowledge, physicians, new medicines, and other marvels of the 20th century. I know there will always be pros and cons about medical treatments and such, but I made the choices that were in my best interests and necessary for me at the time. I do myself and my family the favor of not being too critical about these past decisions.

I truly feel that my medical caregivers came through for me and were instrumental in my surviving breast cancer. I also believe that my emotional caregivers are equally responsible for helping me through a great deal of the physical and mental trauma. They taught me what I needed to know, not only to prolong my life, but to have a better quality of life. And, also, I give myself credit for listening to the right people and trusting my own instincts.

I never thought about having breast cancer, or any kind of cancer for that matter. I guess I thought I was sort of indestructable. I really was totally unprepared, both physically and mentally, for what happened to me in 1989. It was a tremendous shock! But it didn't take me long to learn that I had to play the hand I was dealt and I had to play to win. I must say that I didn't play that hand alone, and I haven't come this far without the help of some very wonderful people. I'm not perfect. I have bad habits as well as good ones. I have made many mistakes during my life, and learned from them. They say you "live and learn"—and I certainly am doing just that.

There is no way on the face of the Earth to put a cost on the pain and suffering my family and I have experienced as a result of cancer. Before 1989, none of us knew anything about a mastectomy, a prosthesis, lymphedema sleeves, chemotherapy drugs, or radiation. But, by the same token, there is no way to put a price on the knowledge and experience we have gained as a result of my having had breast cancer. It really is true what they say about the whole family being affected by cancer and not just the person who actually has the disease. We have all learned extremely valuable and lasting lessons about ourselves and life.

Now I want to put cancer in the past and look forward to better times. It would be humanly impossible to ever forget that I am a breast cancer survivor! That goes without saying. I just want to look ahead to a future filled with all kinds of wonderful surprises, good health, happiness, love, and even *fun*! You know—all the good stuff. I want to travel and see lots of beautiful places and meet lots of interesting

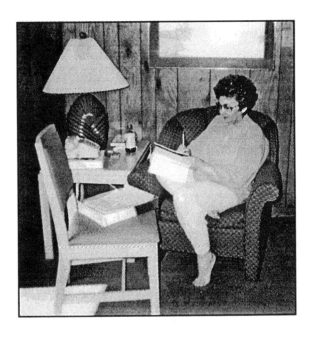

Norma Suzette Jones working on this book at North Myrtle Beach. "We listened to our collection of tapes—and the ocean—while we worked. It was wonderful! When we traveled to the beach to work on the book, we took the word processor, Allie's oxygen tank, and my arm pump. We really did take nearly everything but the kitchen sink!"

people.

I don't simply want to live. I want to *live*! I want to be there for the people who need me and help and support *them* through thick and thin. I want to feel and love and be loved and just be me. I want to laugh and cry and play with my grandchildren and cook turkey for Thanksgiving and wrap gifts at Christmas and celebrate birthdays. I want to talk and listen and smile and get a good night's sleep. I want to pick blackberries and watch the fire in the fireplace and walk in the sand beside the ocean on a hot, hot day. I want to ponder mysteries and give someone a hug and hold something small in my hand that's shiny and beautiful.

I want to do all these things and a zillion more. I understand now that it's not big or grand things that make up the threads of life, but simple, everyday things. Of course, we need the great big events in our lives, too, but to me, it's the little, common things we do without thinking that are the most important threads in the golden fabric of our lives. These sturdy golden threads, made of experience and memories, are the fabric of life that is strong enough to withstand rips and pliable enough to hold more. And, occasionally, a rare sparkling gem of a memory is added for endurance and beauty.

Norma Suzette Jones

Facing Forward: Allie Fair

As I journey forward, I hope to enhance my health and enrich my life. I hope to experience peace, love, and serenity—and to make the personal choices that are right for me.

I feel that my cancer experience was a message for me to change—to change the way I saw myself and the way I saw others. I had to decide what really mattered. I know I will continue to have "ups and downs" like everyone else, but overall, I want to feel good about the way I do things. I hope to find new meaning in all I undertake. I want to enjoy each day as it comes. I want to be able to look at a problem as a challenge, and to be able to turn a crisis into an opportunity. I want to make the world a better place in which to live. I want to enhance my relationships with others, and respect my fellow survivors and their points of view.

I will continue to set goals and have priorities, but no longer feel that I have to be "Superwoman." Instead, I will choose to be *me*. I will still have the qualities that made me a caring mother and a good friend. These qualities have not changed because of cancer. I will still have the same values, interests, and concerns. I will still have the same needs as before—plus new needs: the need to be myself, the need to inspire others, and the need to receive encouragement from others.

There will continue to be moments that I feel that I am on the edge of a cliff, but I hope these moments

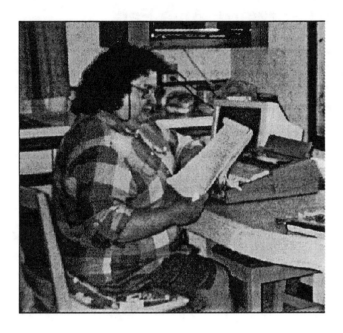

Allie Fair Sawyer writing at the word processor in North Myrtle Beach. "Although we had to have help to get our writing tools and equipment to the beach, feeding the sea gulls was excellent therapy—and it was a lot of fun."

will be fewer and farther between as I strive to return to a normal life.

Surviving is more than reaching a certain stage and feeling that my accomplishment is complete. Surviving is a continuous journey of healing and growing. It's a new way of living!

I will be open to God's guidance and strive to have

a purpose-filled life. As I build my sand castles, I will try to give them a rock foundation. I will strive to add new dimensions to my future. I feel if I live to win in life, I will win. I am looking forward to the future with HOPE.

Allie Fair Sawyer

Notes:

Notes:

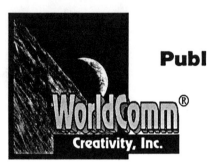